P9-DTT-154

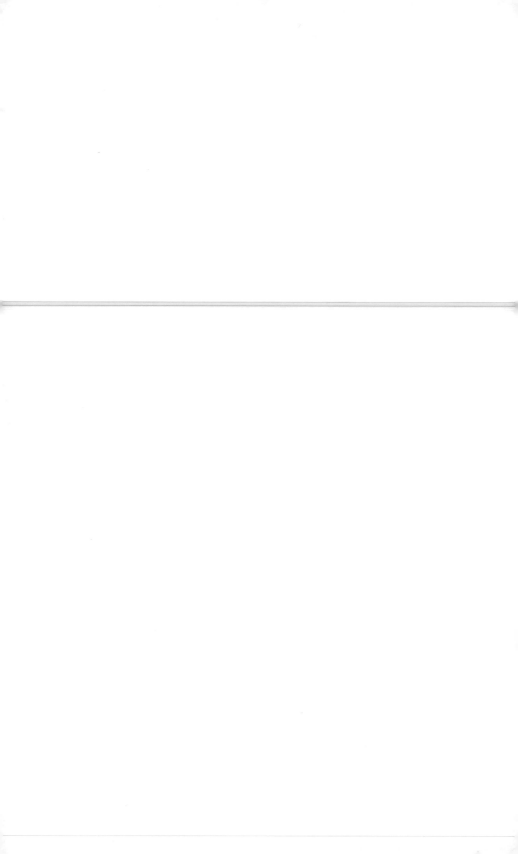

PLANNED BULLYHOOD

The Truth Behind the Headlines about
the Planned Parenthood Funding Battle
with Susan G. Komen for the Cure

KAREN HANDEL

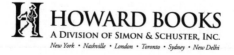

HOWARD BOOKS
A DIVISION OF SIMON & SCHUSTER, INC.
New York · Nashville · London · Toronto · Sydney · New Delhi

Howard Books
A Division of Simon & Schuster, Inc.
1230 Avenue of the Americas
New York, NY 10020

First Howard Books hardcover edition September 2012

Scripture quotations taken from THE HOLY BIBLE, NEW INTERNATIONAL VERSION®, NIV®. Copyright © 1973, 1978, 1984 by Biblica US, Inc.®. Used by permission.

HOWARD and colophon are trademarks of Simon & Schuster, Inc.

For information about special discounts for bulk purchases, please contact Simon & Schuster Special Sales at 1-866-506-1949 or business@simonandschuster.com.

The Simon & Schuster Speakers Bureau can bring authors to your live event. For more information or to book an event, contact the Simon & Schuster Speakers Bureau at 1-866-248-3049 or visit our website at www.simonspeakers.com.

Designed by Jaime Putorti

Manufactured in the United States of America

10   9   8   7   6   5   4   3   2   1

Library of Congress Cataloging-in-Publication Data

Handel, Karen.
    Planned bullyhood : the truth behind the headlines about the Planned Parenthood funding battle with Susan G. Komen for the Cure / Karen Handel.
       p.   cm.
    Includes bibliographical references.
    1. Planned Parenthood Federation of America.   2. Susan G. Komen Breast Cancer Foundation.   3. Handel, Karen.   4. Birth control clinics—United States—Finance.   5. Breast—Cancer—United States.   6. Women's health services—United States—Finance.   7. Abortion services—United States—Finance.   8. Poor women—Services for—United States.   I. Title.
HQ766.5.U5H345 2012
363.9'60973—dc23   2012022884

ISBN 978-1-4516-9794-0
ISBN 978-1-4516-9796-4 (ebook)

This book is dedicated to anyone who has ever been bullied for doing the right thing. In standing up for what you believe, you might not endear yourself to some, but who cares, they don't define you; you do. Have faith—God has a plan, even if it's a mystery to you.

Contents

PLANNED BULLYHOOD

Introduction

On February 2, 2012, Andrea Mitchell of NBC interviewed the head of Susan G. Komen for the Cure, Nancy Brinker. Komen is the world's leading breast cancer organization, a highly regarded institution dedicated to breast cancer education and research with just one mission: to end breast cancer forever.

Nancy founded the organization in 1982 following the death of her sister, Susan G. Komen, from breast cancer. Before she died, Suzy made a request of her sister: do something about breast cancer. Nancy promised that she would and has dedicated her life to keeping that promise to her sister. Komen was born out of that promise—and today, Komen's Race for the Cure and its pink paraphernalia are well-known to most Americans. Thanks to Nancy, dramatic progress has been made in the fight against this disease. Her efforts have literally saved the lives of tens of thousands of women.

And now Brinker was on the air, fighting for the organization's life—for her life's work.

Mitchell, an ardent liberal and breast cancer survivor, was enraged because Komen had decided in December to end its grants to Planned Parenthood Federation of America.

Planned Parenthood, most in the media, liberal interest

groups, and Democratic politicians said Komen's decision was political. It was not; it was an economic one—made in the best interest of Komen and, more important, the women that Komen serves. In fact, Nancy had once been a member of a local Planned Parenthood board and was a former honoree of the organization. She had no ax to grind with Planned Parenthood. But Komen, like most nonprofits, was being affected by the economic downturn. Komen's donors were demanding that grants be as effective as possible. Komen's board of directors was insisting on real, measurable results and even higher standards of excellence. The grants to Planned Parenthood—about $700,000 in 2011, or less than one-tenth of one percent of Planned Parenthood's $1 billion annual budget—were not high-quality grants. Planned Parenthood didn't provide mammograms. Their educational programs were duplicative and there was virtually no way to determine what, if any, tangible, meaningful results were achieved. The decision to stop the Planned Parenthood grants had been months, even years, in the making.

Komen's decision to transition out of the Planned Parenthood grants—to become neutral in the divisive debate on abortion—unleashed a firestorm from the left. The left had decided that Republicans and conservatives were fighting a "war on women"—and, they said, Komen was part of that war. Never mind that Komen's entire mission was breast cancer—not politics, and certainly not abortion. People of every political belief and party had worn the pink shirts, walked with pink boas, and displayed the pink ribbons that have become synonymous with Komen and the fight against breast cancer. To Planned Parenthood and its opportunistic friends in the White House and Congress, daring to walk away would not be tolerated.

Planned Parenthood *was* women, according to those on the left. For Planned Parenthood, there was no such thing as neutral. You were either with them or against them. And anybody who didn't actively support Planned Parenthood was the enemy and had to be destroyed—including a nonpartisan breast cancer foundation doing great work.

Mitchell had a special dog in this fight. She's a major advocate for Planned Parenthood and calls it a noble organization.[1] She and MSNBC had stacked the guest list that morning on behalf of Planned Parenthood. First, Planned Parenthood president Cecile Richards had appeared to announce that her organization was "very shocked and really surprised" by the decision—which struck me as less than genuine since they had known about the decision for weeks and the two organizations had agreed to share messaging and not go to the press. We believed we were working toward an amicable split—right up to the day Cecile deliberately lit the fuse with the media. Then Mitchell linked up Planned Parenthood allies Senator Barbara Boxer (D-CA) and Senator Patty Murray (D-WA) to do a postmortem.

Mitchell came out with both guns blazing. "The storm has exploded," she chided Nancy. "I have to tell you this is shocking for a lot of your longtime supporters." She then explained to Nancy that she'd been at the gym that morning and was confronted by a woman who told her she'd never wear a Komen T-shirt again. "How could this have taken place?" Mitchell demanded.

From the outset of the interview, it was clear: the media, the Obama administration, its Democratic allies in Congress, and Planned Parenthood were working together in a coordinated attack on Komen.

And that's when Andrea Mitchell mentioned my name.

"The fact is," said Mitchell, "a lot of people are tracing this back. My colleague, Lisa Myers, reporting last night on *Nightly News,* a lot of people are tracing this back to what some found [to be] the surprising hiring of Karen Handel, who ran for governor. We've seen her statements and her strong support. She said when she was running for office, 'I am staunchly and unequivocally pro-life. Let me be clear, since I am pro-life, I do not support the mission of Planned Parenthood.' So, the question is, for a bipartisan organization such as yours, which has a broad-based advisory group, why hire a key staff person who is so strongly, fiercely identified against Planned Parenthood, one of your grantees?"[2]

And suddenly, I was the focus of the fury of the left.

———

I never anticipated many of the events in my life—including writing this book. To a certain extent, all of us have a desire to speak our truth, and I am no different. But *this* is different.

This is the story of how one of the least controversial organizations in America—an organization dedicated solely to eradicating breast cancer—became a target of the left for simply trying to do the right thing for its mission.

This is the recounting of what really happened when the big pink bus collided head-on with the political machine of one of the left's most ruthless enforcers; of how individuals who were simply trying to do their jobs became grist for the politics of personal destruction.

This is the story of how Planned Parenthood, in partnership with the liberal establishment, made Komen pay for daring to put its mission above the ideology of the almighty left. Planned Parenthood became the left's ultimate tip of the spear in an election-year battle to maintain the White House, willing to destroy anyone or any organization that might get in the way.

When I joined Komen, the last thing I wanted was controversy. I'd already had my share of it. I believed in Komen's mission, and I wanted Komen's donors to know that their dollars were being invested in the most effective, impactful way possible to fulfill Komen's reason for being: "fighting every minute of every day to finish what we started and achieve our vision of a world without breast cancer."

Yes, I am pro-life, but that had nothing to do with my work at Komen. Komen was about ending breast cancer, not abortion. Ironically, when I ran for governor of Georgia, I was the only Republican candidate *not* endorsed by Georgia Right to Life—they'd been too busy calling me "desperate" and "barren." My position on Planned Parenthood's abortion services hadn't been central to my campaign. I was even attacked by my Republican opponents in the gubernatorial primaries for not doing more to stop the distribution of federal grants to Planned Parenthood during my time as a county commission chairman.

I was at Komen for one reason and one reason only: to help them in the fight against breast cancer. I was hired in April 2011.

My job was senior vice president of public policy, and as part of that job, I was tasked with identifying options to disengage from Planned Parenthood.

For at least a decade, Komen had been considering whether to end funding to Planned Parenthood. The organization had been dealing with the backlash from pro-life conservatives because of its grants to the country's largest abortion provider. In 2011, the criticism intensified as Planned Parenthood became mired in scandal. A New Jersey Planned Parenthood clinic was mixed up in a sex trafficking incident caught on tape. The U.S. House of Representatives had voted to stop all federal funding to the abortion provider. And, several states had taken action to prohibit funding to the group. Komen was facing boycotts from Catholics, Baptists, and numerous pro-life groups. Corporate sponsors were withdrawing, not wanting to be associated with controversy. Race participants were pulling out. Komen's local affiliates were frustrated, and their fund-raising was being affected. Add to this Komen's own mounting public relations issues and declining revenues, and something had to give. In late fall of 2011, Senator Marco Rubio (R-FL) withdrew as honorary co-chairman of Komen's Palm Beach event after backlash from his participation in a Komen race and a call from his bishop. Weeks later, LifeWay Christian Resources of the Southern Baptist Convention recalled its pink Bible, which had benefited Komen. That was the last straw.

Nancy, along with Komen president Liz Thompson and others, was weary of the "pink" being tarnished by Planned Parenthood's controversies and wanted Komen out of the middle of the pro-life/abortion debate. It was not our issue. It had become a major distraction, sucking up manpower and putting a damper on fund-raising. We were a breast cancer organization, and we couldn't afford to offend either side, particularly on the basis of crappy grants to Planned Parenthood.

I use the word *crappy* advisedly. It's not even my word, actually—it's Liz's, her way of describing low-quality grants that were not particularly impactful. Komen already had a major initiative under way to revamp its granting model to focus more on outcomes. There were only nineteen Planned Parenthood grants in sixteen communities, and most were viewed as poor-quality grants delivering minimal results. The total amount Planned Parenthood received was about $680,000. That's less than one percent of Komen's total $93 million community grant portfolio. Ending the grants would be controversial, but there would be no negative impact on the women Komen serves. Planned Parenthood would be disappointed—even angry—but with its $1 billion budget, the grants were inconsequential to its work.

So Komen made a rational, reasonable decision: implement a new community granting strategy that would drive better health outcomes for women—and, in doing so, move to neutral ground in the culture wars by severing ties with Planned Parenthood. This, in turn, would eliminate a major headache while redirecting the dollars to programs that could better serve women and open a new, robust fund-raising channel.

In mid-December 2011, Komen and Planned Parenthood agreed to work together on messaging and agreed not to proactively go to the press or ambush one another—a "gentle-ladies agreement," if you will. Cecile Richards and company would soon violate this agreement. Both organizations acknowledged that a media firestorm was in no one's best interest. Komen expanded its already significant stable of star consultants, which included Morris + King, Ogilvy's Brendan Daly—former communications director for Nancy Pelosi, and who had served alongside another former Pelosi staffer, Cecile Richards—and Republican strategist Ari Fleischer, adding Democratic insider Hilary Rosen of the high-powered, left-leaning firm SKDKnickerbocker. Rosen was to be the Planned Parenthood liaison and manage the left.

Yet, despite the agreement not to go to the press, six weeks later Planned Parenthood did just that and unleashed an attack so vicious and so elegantly executed that I could see only one logical conclusion: it was premeditated, coordinated, and precisely timed. It involved the highest levels of the liberal establishment, including the head of the Democratic National Committee, Congresswoman Debbie Wasserman Schultz. It included the Obama administration, which was able to use Komen to distract from its burgeoning problem with Catholic voters over contraception mandates. The firestorm put Komen at the center of the "war on women," being pushed by Democrats. And Planned Parenthood's attack was executed with ruthless precision, despite Komen having brought on board the high-powered Democratic strategist Hilary Rosen. I became the eye of that storm.

It was a battle of wills.

And Komen lost.

After just three days, following hysterical cries that "Komen was abandoning women"—fueled by a brutal social media campaign and blatantly biased mainstream press—Komen capitulated and reversed course. Komen's surrender was even encouraged by conservative mainstays like Karl Rove.

That was Friday. I resigned the next Tuesday.

The left declared victory. They said I was a right-wing Trojan horse and that Komen's decision to drop Planned Parenthood had been part of my nefarious plan to take over the organization and turn it into an instrument of the pro-life movement.

Meanwhile, the pro-life community hailed me as a hero, standing up for my views on the sanctity of human life. Yes, I was and am staunchly pro-life, but portraying me as their hero wasn't accurate, either. I believed—and still believe—that breast cancer is not about ideology. Yet when Komen gave up on being neutral and caved to the mafia-style tactics of Planned Parenthood and the left, Komen made it about ideology.

Two weeks after I left Komen—two weeks after the Planned Parenthood thugs had waged their merciless war against Komen—I received disturbing information. Komen was message-shopping yet another new spin on the decision—an appropriate decision that had now been hijacked for political purposes. Thousands were being surveyed—being asked to rate me as favorable or unfavorable and to evaluate several positioning statements, including: "We have made mistakes, which we thoroughly regret. The person at the center of this controversy, Komen Senior Vice President, has left the organization . . ."

I hadn't joined Komen to be at the eye of any storm. I found myself there nonetheless.

Why did Planned Parenthood break its word, go to the press, and ambush Komen? Why did Planned Parenthood purposely set out to destroy Komen over dollars that were clearly insignificant, given its $1 billion budget? How did Planned Parenthood—along with the media and leaders of the liberal establishment—have inside information about Komen's decision? Planned Parenthood had six weeks to plan its devastating shakedown operation. The timing was specific—timing that, by "chance," was the most advantageous for the Obama administration. Why did Democratic National Committee (DNC) chairman Wasserman Schultz's office place a call to Komen the week before Planned Parenthood went nuclear, asking Nancy Brinker to call Wasserman Schultz immediately—only to delay the supposedly urgent call until the following week, to the very day that the press and Planned Parenthood pushed the button? Hilary Rosen's firm includes several former high-ranking Obama staffers, including Anita Dunn, who had served as the White House communications director. The firm also has strong ties to Planned Parenthood, even handling some of its public relations. Did this conflict play a role? What about Brendan Daly? He worked with Cecile Richards in Pelosi's office. Were these all just insignificant coincidences?

The episode has left the iconic breast cancer organization reeling. In attempting to walk away from Planned Parenthood, Komen unwittingly unleashed the fury of abortion rights fanatics, the wrath of Democrats, and the indignation of the liberal-leaning media. Komen ignited a battle in which it became collateral damage in a larger election-year contest between liberals and conservatives for the souls (and votes!) of women and the nation's conscience—with "women's health" becoming the rallying cry for the liberals.

The Komen incident also exposed an underlying and disturbing truth: Planned Parenthood and its allies are the worst kind of bullies. They were willing to do almost anything to advance their political agenda and ensure the continued flow of nearly $1.5 million dollars a day in government money to Planned Parenthood's coffers.

That's why I left Komen: to be free to tell the full and unadulterated truth—not attributed to unnamed sources and distorted by media assumptions and outright lies. The truth can be uncomfortable and even hurtful, but that is no reason to avoid telling it. This is the true story of Komen's real motives, Planned Parenthood's tactics, and my role in it all. The tyrannical leftist infrastructure—Planned Parenthood, Obama, the DNC, the media—joined forces to conduct a crushing shakedown of Komen and bully it into submission. Planned Parenthood was Obama's consigliere and the DNC's enforcer. It was Planned Bullyhood. It *was* planned. And it *was* bullying. And the bullying won't stop until it is exposed—and we stand up to it.

1

Trojan Horse?
Pro-Life Hero?
I'm Just Karen

Liberals say I am a Trojan horse for Republicans, pro-lifers, or the Catholic Church—or, if you're reading MoveOn.org, all three. They say I used deceit to advance my personal pro-life beliefs, my Catholic faith, and my politics at the expense of Komen.

Many conservatives said I was a pro-life hero. It's true that I am pro-life, but I'm no hero.

I'm just Karen—a rather ordinary individual who found herself at the center of an extraordinary series of events. I've never let others define who I am, and I'm not about to now. I embrace God's plan for me—while wondering at the meaning and irony of the many things that have happened in my life.

———

Like most people, my views have been shaped by my experiences, events around me, and those individuals who have been influential in my life.

When I was eight years old, my brother and I learned that we were going to have a sister or brother. I was so excited. But Mom and Dad didn't seem so excited. Mom was sick—really sick. Dad was anxious. Looking back, I'm sure my parents knew early on that something was wrong.

Abortion was not yet widely legal in the United States, but it was certainly available. Now, I'm not suggesting that my parents ever considered this—just that there were options. We weren't wealthy by any stretch. My father was a county worker. The thought of the emotional and financial strain of a child with serious, possibly permanent health issues had to have been daunting. Regardless, my parents did everything they could to bring that baby safely into this world no matter what the future held.

In early March 1970, my baby sister Jennifer arrived. Something was very wrong. She was born with a congenital medical condition called esophageal atresia. In Jennifer's case, it was one of the most serious forms of the condition—rather than the esophagus failing to close properly, Jennifer was missing virtually all of her esophagus. Her chances of survival were slim.

She spent most of the first two years of her life in the hospital. But thanks to the miracles of medical advancements, the care and expertise of her doctors and nurses, and the prayers of so many, Jennifer's condition was fixed. Today Jennifer is a healthy, successful woman, the mother of my two beautiful nieces. And she is one of the most amazing people I know.

I considered my family religious. We went to church most every Sunday. Yet, as it is with a lot of families in their Sunday best, what was seen from the pews hid the truth of serious troubles at home.

By the time I was in my teens, home was the last place I wanted to be. Not because I was some kind of party girl. To the contrary, I was an excellent student—nearly all As (except for gym, geometry, and that one semester when we had to read *Beowulf*). I didn't want to be home, because I never knew if it was going to be a good day or a bad day.

As I entered my senior year of high school, nearly every day was a bad day, and the others were even worse. Mom's Budweiser-fueled rages were becoming more violent. And I was her target.

I needed a plan that would let me move out as soon as I graduated. I enrolled in a program that allowed me to take my Advanced Placement (AP) classes in the morning and work in the afternoon. I was lucky enough to be hired by our county school superintendent.

Still, I had not given up on my dream of college. No one in my family had a college degree. I was going to be the first. With a good SAT score, good grades, a proven work ethic, and the achievement of being a National Merit Scholarship finalist, I would surely be able to qualify for a scholarship and financial aid to a decent school—if not a great school.

I just needed Dad to complete the financial section of the scholarship and financial aid forms. He refused.

Devastated could not begin to describe how I felt. But, as I had often had to do, and would have to do many more times in my life, I focused on what was ahead and what could be—instead of what was not to be.

In early 1980, after a particularly violent encounter with my mother, I left the house for good. Graduation was still a few months away, and I was able to stay with a family in the neighborhood. I finished school and graduated with my class that May.

Without scholarships or financial aid, going to college fulltime was not an option. But, then, it wasn't an option for a lot of eighteen-year-olds. So I got a job—as a clerk typist with the American Association of Retired Persons (AARP)—and enrolled in evening and Saturday classes at the local community college, and then later at the University of Maryland's University College.

That November, I would cast my first ballot for president of the United States of America—for Ronald Reagan. I believed in Ronald Reagan and his words of optimism about America's best days not being behind her. Or maybe it was just that I *needed* to believe him; to believe in a country that was so great, with so many opportunities that the future was bright—even for a young girl like me. All I had to do was work hard and I could do and be whatever I chose. Because if America's best days were ahead, that meant mine could be, too. My conservative core was set.

The next two years were filled with work and school. I left AARP after about two years for a bigger paycheck at a law firm. I continued my college at night, concentrating on accounting courses.

On a whim, I applied for a position in the Washington, D.C., government affairs office for Hallmark Cards.

A Central Figure Enters My Life

At this point, I had been in the work world for a few years, but I was still very rough around the edges and anything but polished—except for my way-too-long nails, which were painted bright red, especially for this job interview.

My interview was with Rae Forker Evans, Hallmark's vice president of national affairs. Still today, she and I laugh about this first meeting.

With an incredulous look, Rae asked, "Can you really type with those things?"

Trying to be confident, but revealing the chip on my shoulder, I blurted: "How many words would you like?" As soon as I said the words I wanted to take them back. Who was I kidding? This woman was successful—she was somebody in Washington. She needed an educated, put-together executive assistant who could interact smoothly with members of Congress and other high-level corporate executives. I left thinking there was no way I'd get this job.

A few days later, Rae called and offered me the position—at a salary nearly three thousand dollars below what I was making. I took the job anyway. Somehow I just knew that I had to work for this woman.

And Rae Forker Evans would be a defining person in my life.

Rae saw things in me that I had never seen in myself. She gave me opportunities that few others would have. She was tough and demanding, but fair. Rae is a powerhouse—a true trailblazer.

Rae ran the public policy office for Hallmark. I was her executive assistant, but in a three-person office and especially one headed by Rae Evans, you had better be ready and able to do a lot more than type and answer phones. Before too long, I was planning events on Capitol Hill, coordinating the attendance of members of Congress at Hallmark events, doing research, analyzing legislation, and covering Hill hearings. I even attended my first Republican National Convention and volunteered on my first political campaign.

Ironically enough, it was through politics that I first became involved in the fight against breast cancer.

Again, it was Rae who made it happen.

Working with the Quayles

A few months into the Bush-Quayle administration, in early 1989, Marilyn Quayle, wife of Vice President Dan Quayle, decided that breast cancer awareness was an issue she would champion, and she needed someone to coordinate her activities. Rae suggested me. I was offered the position. At first, I wasn't sure I wanted it. The truth was that I was still unsure of myself. Would I really fit in? This was the *White House.* But with her typical tact, Rae made a suggestion: "You're taking the job at the White House," she said. "This is nonnegotiable."

That first day, I passed through the guard shack and onto the grounds of the White House. I had never even been on a tour of the White House, let alone imagined that I would work there. I made my way to the second floor of the Old Executive Office

Building next door—excited but nervous. Once again, I had been given the opportunity of a lifetime.

My job was everything I hoped it would be—challenging and exciting. After a year or so, I was promoted to deputy chief of staff.

I wrote speeches, handled constituent services, coordinated breast cancer awareness events, and served as Marilyn's liaison with various organizations, including the Susan G. Komen Foundation, as it was called then. Vice President and Mrs. Quayle agreed to be the honorary chairpersons of Komen's signature event, the Race for the Cure in Washington, D.C. It was through this event that I first met Nancy Brinker, Komen's founder.

Marilyn Quayle's work was more than just speeches and races. She was the National Cancer Institute's spokesperson for the National Cancer Summits and played an instrumental role in the establishment of the National Institutes of Health's Office of Research on Women's Health. She was an active member of a coalition that included Komen, the American Cancer Society, other organizations, and congressional wives to get Congress to officially designate October as National Breast Cancer Awareness Month.

Marilyn Tucker Quayle made a significant, lasting impact in the fight against breast cancer, and in many ways, her contributions have been overlooked.

Marilyn made a deep impact on me, too. While I believed that abortion was wrong, it was more because of my faith; I hadn't really considered what it meant to be "pro-life." Marilyn Quayle is staunchly pro-life, and her views on family made a particular impression on me. This was the time of *Murphy Brown,* when Vice President Quayle was vilified for suggesting that the CBS sitcom's title character, played by Candice Bergen, was symptomatic of a broader societal acceptance of unwed motherhood and a diminished role for fathers. I never thought that his comments or their beliefs had anything to do with single mothers. Rather, the Quayles saw a trivialization of parenthood and, specifically, of fatherhood. It made me think about what I wanted for my own future, my deep desire for a family and to be a mother someday.

In my life, I have been blessed to cross paths with several extraordinary individuals. Marilyn Quayle is one of them. As a young staffer, it was disheartening and disillusioning to see the cruelty of the press and liberals toward the Quayles. But Marilyn showed me that no one—not your opponents and not the press—defines who you are. We define ourselves through our actions and our convictions. And one must be steadfast in those convictions—as a person, and even more so in public office. How could I know that one day I would experience some of the same difficult treatment?

I was honored to be part of their team. But after seeing all that the Quayles had gone through, I knew for certain that a political career was not for me; I was headed to the corporate world.

Finding the One

During that time, I met Steve—the man who would become the love of my life. Like Rae, Steve saw in me things that I didn't see in myself—he had a way of bringing out a different me, a better me. I was used to fending for myself. I had to be tough, sometimes overly so. But with Steve I wasn't afraid to show a softer side, to let my guard down. He was spontaneous; I hated surprises. He was the cool and calm to my fiery, sometimes hot-headed nature. We were married the Saturday after the November 1992 presidential election, in which George H. W. Bush and Dan Quayle lost their bid for a second term to Bill Clinton. God really does have a way of balancing things out.

Following My Career Goal

After the White House, I landed a job as the director of public and media relations for the Fur Information Council of America, the innocuously named trade association for the fur retail industry. This might seem like a crazy move to some, but it made perfect sense to me. My career goal was to head a major company's public affairs team. I needed to get a tough, controversial issue under my belt, and I needed media experience. This job gave me both. By 1992, People for the Ethical Treatment of Animals—or PETA—had turned radical, escalating its attacks on the fur industry and fur wearers. My job was to represent the industry with the press and create PR and promotional programs.

Georgia Becomes Home

In late 1993, Steve was offered a promotion—in Atlanta. So, early the next year, off we went. If we didn't like it, we could always move back.

For me, moving to Georgia was a little like Cinderella going to the ball—and I knew I had found home. We could suddenly afford our dream house in a great neighborhood close to the best schools. And the timing was perfect to start a family. So, we bought the dream house—complete with the perfect backyard.

By the end of the year, it was time for a new opportunity. Working out of the house was convenient, but I needed to get engaged in the community—to build a professional network in Georgia. When I went to work for the accounting firm of KPMG, yet another extraordinary individual entered my life— Neal Purcell. Still, KPMG would be an interim stop for me. My plan in the next two years was to be the head of public affairs for a major company and become a mom. Just like Rae.

After two years with KPMG, there was still no baby. Each month—despite doctors' visits, and hoping and praying for a family—it was the same: heartbreak.

But on the career front, things were right on track. Through KPMG I met Glen Bradley, CEO of CIBA Vision, a global eye care company and then a division of Novartis. Glen hired me as the company's global head of communications and public affairs—with a twist. I reported to the chief financial officer, who taught me how to translate financial statements and gave me a deep understanding of budgeting—skills that would later be important.

My career was going as planned. Steve was doing great. Life was really good—except still no baby.

I traveled a lot with my job at CIBA Vision. After a few years, and despite achieving the position I had always wanted, I remained unfulfilled. What I wanted most was to be a mom. I figured that a job with less travel and less stress might make a difference, since nothing else seemed to. I left CIBA Vision to become president and CEO of the North Fulton Chamber of Commerce.

A Different Life

I went to work getting to know the chamber's members, programs, and finances.

It would take only a few months for me to discover that the Chamber's audits were fraudulent, our finances in disarray. The Chamber was on the brink of bankruptcy. The "trusted" finance director had been embezzling for nearly seven years.

It was a mess. It was embarrassing. Some wanted to keep the situation quiet, but I was convinced that the best approach was to be open and honest—and prosecute the finance director to the fullest extent of the law. If the board wanted to sweep it under the rug, so be it, but they would do it over my resignation. Fortunately, I didn't have to resign. The case was turned over to the county district attorney, and eventually the finance director pleaded guilty to five counts of theft by taking and three counts of forgery in the first degree.[1]

I was determined that this chamber would not fold under my leadership.

Over the course of the following year, thanks to the support of the community and the members, the debt was nearly paid off and the Chamber was back on track.

━━━━━━━

Personally, I was a wreck. The past eight years had been the most difficult of my life—and of Steve's, too. The emotional pain of not being able to conceive was beginning to take a serious toll. We had even tried fertility treatments, hoping and praying for a miracle. I put on the "happy face" and did what I had to do each day. But, every month—month after month—I was devastated. Our friends were having babies. I didn't begrudge them, but why them and not us? I couldn't bring myself to attend baby showers. News stories about abortion or some mother who callously threw her newborn into a trash bin or even just the sight of a mother and baby made my sorrow deeper and more palpable.

Steve and I had to make a decision—for the sake of our marriage; for my sake. Do we cross the bridge to a life without children of our own and trust that God will give us the opportunity for a different life—one that could still be happy and fulfilling—or do we stay in a place so filled with pain that it is tearing us apart and destroying us both emotionally? We crossed the bridge—together, with Steve holding my hand the entire way—trusting that God would indeed "make the rough places smooth" and that a new path was being prepared for us (from Isaiah 42:16 and 40:4).

Out of this very personal, painful struggle, my pro-life beliefs were deepened. Little did I know that our inability to have children would later become the focal point of a political attack that would put me right in the middle of the abortion debate.

Running for Office

As Steve and I adjusted to a different kind of life together, another opportunity came my way—one that would take our lives down a new path, a path we never could have predicted. This time, local Republicans wanted me to run for public office.

Rob Simms recruited me. He was chief of staff to the Fulton County commission chairman and deeply involved in county politics. We were having lunch, discussing the upcoming county commission races and the business community's perspectives. After throwing out the names of various possibilities, Rob got to his point: he and others wanted me to run.

That night, I laughed when I told Steve about it. Steve, though, didn't think it was funny at all. He said he could see me doing it.

I ran for District 2 county commission in Fulton County, a majority-Democratic county. My opponent was a longtime Democratic politician who had spent twenty years on the Atlanta City Council and just lost a close race for mayor of Atlanta. Our race came down to a seasoned Democratic politician against the "girl" from the fast-growing Republican end of the county.

I lost by fewer than 5,000 votes out of nearly 200,000 cast.

I was disappointed, but as is my nature, I focused on what was ahead. Georgia now had a Republican governor. Sonny Perdue overcame a massive fund-raising deficit to be elected Georgia's first Republican governor in 130 years. I still had my job at the Chamber, and Steve and I were off to Hawaii to celebrate our tenth wedding anniversary.

An Opportunity with the New Governor

Governor Perdue shocked me by tapping me to be his deputy chief of staff. I left the Chamber and joined his administration in January 2003.

Once again, God was balancing the bitter of the past year—and a new path for Steve and me lay ahead.

Being part of Sonny's administration was as challenging as it was exciting. My role was less political and focused more on constituent services, citizen liaison, and supporting the chief of staff in running the day-to-day operations of the governor's office.

Sonny was a man of deep faith, and he never hesitated to show his faith in how he lived and governed. A few years later, when he held a day of prayer during Georgia's worst drought in decades, many ridiculed him for turning to God. What I saw was a man who had the courage to draw on his faith—a leader who embraced the role of God in our lives and our country. Sonny helped me understand that faith could—and should—be part of any leader's decision making. This was an important lesson in leadership that I carry with me today. Oh, it rained!

Just five months into Governor Perdue's administration, the county commission chairman resigned unexpectedly. I had not given any thought to running for office again, and certainly not so soon. But as I've come to learn, you don't get to pick the timing in politics; politics picks the timing for you.

This time it was a real campaign. Rob Simms was on board. Nick Ayers, who had just come off of Perdue's winning campaign and would go on to become the head of the Republican Governors Association, was the campaign manager.

My toughest opponent was a former commissioner, and I got my first taste of the malicious side of politics. For the first time in my life, I was accused of being a racist. There are a lot of ways to describe me but racist is certainly not among them.

I won the race with a large majority. Suddenly I was chairman of the county commission—the first woman chairman—for a county with nearly one million people, Georgia's largest and most populated.

If the chamber was a mess when I joined, Fulton County was a disaster. A $100 million budget deficit. A proposed massive property tax increase to fill the gap. A bickering, divisive commission controlled by Democrats. Long-running allegations of corruption—several commissioners had even gone to jail in recent years.

I had pledged to be a leader who could get things done—no tax increases; strong ethics.

First up: a new budget. My chief of staff and I went to work.

The Democratic commissioners were irate. Who did I think I was? They had a budget. The budget sessions were contentious, as was every meeting that followed. I stood firm. Took their insults. Made my case—in the media and directly to the people of the county. And finally, after some losses, some compromises, and an effective parliamentary strategy, the budget passed. The deficit was closed. The budget was balanced. There was *no* tax increase that year.

I would have to beat back tax increases each year. And somehow, with the help of a great team and the support of Fulton County citizens, we balanced the county budget without tax increases each and every year under my tenure as chairman. We even implemented one of the strongest ethics codes of any county in the country.

A few months into my term, an audit revealed that $7 million was missing from an account the county sheriff controlled. Completely gone.

The Fulton County sheriff was Jackie Barrett. She was the first female African American sheriff in the country and a National Sheriff of the Year honoree.

All I could think was, *Here we go again.*

Two things were clear. First, $7 million in taxpayer funds had been invested with the sheriff's friends and political cronies, almost certainly in violation of the law, and now it was missing. Second, Barrett had to go.

But I had no authority to remove her. She was an elected official in her own right—and a powerful one. The public was demanding action. The press wanted to know where I stood.

Rob Simms, who continued as a close confidant and advisor, said with his usual directness: hold a press conference today and call for her immediate resignation.

As I would do many times in the coming years, I called Mike Bowers—a friend, a supporter, one of the smartest, toughest people I know, and Georgia's former attorney general. He didn't tell me what to do; that's not his way. He simply said: "There are two types of elected officials: those that become aware of a problem and do nothing—they become part of the problem; and those who stand up and do whatever it takes to fix the problem. Karen, you have to decide which one you are going to be."

I knew what kind of elected official I wanted to be. I knew what I had to do.

I asked for Barrett's resignation. When she refused, I pursued every option available. Eventually she stepped down.

There were death threats. Hundreds of emails. Most were supportive, but some were nasty. Some said I was an ambitious politician using trumped-up allegations to advance my own career. Some said I was a racist.

While there was a loud outpouring from the public and the press, my commission colleagues were unusually silent.

The silence from my fellow elected Republicans was most disappointing. This was my first hint that I was not and never would be part of their club, and it would not be the last time I would have to have the guts to stand alone.

My Introduction to Planned Parenthood

My first real "encounter" with Planned Parenthood came in 2004 when I was on the county commission. Numerous items that were considered routine were regularly put on the consent agenda by staff for an en masse vote with no discussion. One of the items was a grant to Planned Parenthood for well-baby and healthy-women programs. I voted yes on the entire package of items. This vote would become campaign fodder in the coming years.

As is the case in states across the country, federal Title X funding passes through the state budget and is allocated to counties with strict state and federal guidelines, and Planned Parenthood was the only contractor to meet the tightly prescribed requirements. Planned Parenthood had been receiving the grants for some time, and these grants were considered noncontroversial. Unfortunately, that's how the issue was viewed then, and I simply missed the item on the agenda.

My vote was not a vote in support of Planned Parenthood or its abortion agenda. It was a vote *for* the scores of other important programs that were part of that consent agenda package. In retrospect, especially knowing what I know now about Planned Parenthood, this was a fight that I should have taken on.

If my vote on the commission would later undermine my pro-life credibility, my tenure as chairman established a track record of strong budget controls and government ethics—and of being an individual more comfortable and adept with policy making and problem solving than with raw politics.

Raw Politics

On January 12, 2007, Steve was holding my hand as we looked out from the dais of Atlanta's Philips Arena. We were taking in the moment. It was a big one. Our family and friends were there. Rae was there. Governor Perdue was about to swear me in as Georgia's first elected Republican secretary of state.

The secretary of state campaign was my first GOP primary fight—and it would be my first conflict with Georgia Right to Life and all-or-nothing pro-lifers.

The previous spring, I had announced my candidacy for secretary of state. Steve and I were already uncertain about running for reelection as commission chairman. That would mean four more years on the commission—and the three years I'd already served felt like one hundred.

Governor Perdue was running for reelection and the lieutenant governor's seat was open. Two candidates had already announced—former Christian Coalition leader Ralph Reed and Casey Cagle, a little-known state senator. Some GOPers grumbled about the field, and my name was floated.

Me? Lieutenant governor? Why me? The only rationale anyone offered was that I could win and I was a woman. That was shallow and insufficient. Sure, I could do the job—that wasn't the issue. For me, being able to win was not enough of a reason to run for any office.

After much contemplation, Steve and I made the decision together: I would run, but not for lieutenant governor—for secretary of state.

State senate majority leader Bill Stephens was already in the race, along with Charlie Bailey, who had run before, and an unknown candidate Eric Martin. Stephens was considered a lock to win the nomination outright. A longtime Georgia legislator, he'd paid his dues. He had the endorsements of nearly every legislator. I was the upstart; an outsider who had not used my time on the county commission to endear myself to the GOP legislative power center. I was written off, with most saying I couldn't raise the money needed and didn't have the guts to go through with it.

They were right about one thing: I did have a hard time raising money. But no one realized that a lack of guts has never been an issue for me.

Stephens quickly proclaimed himself the "true conservative" and tagged me the "liberal woman from Atlanta."

He said I was not pro-life. My vote on the Planned Parenthood grants at Fulton County was his proof.

I finished the primary at 44 percent, against his 33 percent. We headed into the runoff with Stephens pressing the "she's not a conservative" theme harder. Among his supporters, a nasty whisper campaign was pushed on the blogs—speculating that, with no children, Steve and I were actually gay, our marriage a sham.

However, our biggest challenge came not from Stephens himself but from Georgia Right to Life. GRTL said I did not meet its standard of pro-life. Oh, I knew I would have to address the Planned Parenthood grants. But not pro-life? Yes, I supported legislative exceptions in the cases of rape and incest, but how did that make me pro-abortion?

I met with GRTL and laid out my views. Life begins at conception. Abortion is wrong—under any circumstances—but some things are simply impossible to legislate. No statute could contemplate something so horrible, so traumatic as a woman—or a young girl—becoming pregnant as a result of rape or incest. I'd be a champion for the pro-life cause, a female messenger who could address the issue in ways no man ever could. We agreed on 98 percent of the pro-life issues. But GRTL was not persuaded.

Some key supporters suggested that I just check the box for no exceptions. Who would know? The secretary of state had no impact on abortion policy anyway. Now, I was not persuaded.

GRTL did not endorse me.

I won the runoff against Stephens with nearly 57 percent of the vote and went on to win the general election with 54 percent. The hard work of the team—Marty, Michael, Jamie, Robert, and of course Steve and Rob—and the support of the many Georgians who had put their faith in the upstart had paid off.

While I earned a reputation as a tenacious, hardworking candidate, I had also provoked the ire of GRTL and the pro-life establishment. I had dared to defy them.

Working at the Capitol

My first weeks at the Georgia State Capitol following inauguration were exciting—and revealing. I had heard about the "culture" of the capital—deal making, double dealing, partying, womanizing, and just general bad behavior by some. I wanted no part of it and focused on the job.

Our top legislative priority that first year was to secure an added $1 million in our budget for voter education and outreach that was critical to getting Georgia's new voter ID law out of the courts and up and running. We briefed legislators and testified at budget hearings. We cut the budget elsewhere and reassured everyone that these were one-time dollars and not a permanent expansion of the secretary of state agency's budget. We made the point that we had an obligation to communicate the change to the voters. The response was always positive, but I couldn't shake the feeling that the "we've got you covered" replies were more like pats on the head with a silent "Run along now, little girl. We'll take care of things."

When the House released the budget, the funding was not included.

We arranged a meeting with the Speaker of the House Glenn Richardson. Rob and I strategized ahead of time about the tack to take. Sweet and demure? Straightforward and tough? After all of the usual pleasantries, I got down to business. For those who know me, it will come as no surprise that I went with the tough, candid approach. It worked.

By the end of the meeting, we were both laughing, and I learned that there would be times when I had to stake out my ground. He learned—and others did as well—that I was no wilting lily, and I'd face off with him or anyone else if needed.

The funding came through, and with the voter education initiative, the court injunction was lifted. Georgia's voter photo ID law would go into effect and later be upheld by the courts. This would be one of our most important accomplishments.

Over the next two years, I worked to reduce the agency's budget by nearly 20 percent, improve customer service, and prepare our state for the upcoming 2008 presidential elections. Our office also continued to push aggressive election reform, including proof of citizenship and new-voter verification. While the various Republican candidates sought my endorsement as the state's top female elected official, I declined to endorse any candidate. I did not because of my role in administering the elections. It seemed a conflict, and I wanted to give no one the opportunity to question my actions or decisions in what I assumed would be a contentious battle for the White House.

The GOP faithful gave me high marks. Many legislators were less enthusiastic.

My disdain for the atmosphere at the capitol was well-known. I didn't hide it. I didn't even try to hide it. Sordid scandals— womanizing, lobbyist affairs, drunken-driving arrests—were in the news with increasing frequency. And each time, the matter was brushed off. Lobbyist-paid gifts, event tickets, lavish dinners, and trips for legislators were drawing increasing scrutiny and criticism—in the media and from voters.

I couldn't control the ethics rules of the state legislature, but I did control the ethics within the secretary of state's office. My first month in office, we implemented a ban on gifts, abolished the time-honored tradition of nepotism, and even established a one-year cooling-off period during which no former staffer could lobby the agency. And these rules applied to me as well.

I took my job seriously. And, that's what it was for me—my job. I didn't socialize with legislators and I didn't hit the party circuit. When I socialized, I did so with Steve and our friends— most of whom had nothing whatsoever to do with politics.

The Gold Dome was a clique—a good-old-boys club for which groveling to those in power and turning a blind eye to bad behavior were the required dues. For many lobbyists it was the price of doing business. I did not fit in. I did not *want* to fit in.

Running for Governor

Governor Perdue was term-limited, creating an open seat for governor in 2010. Insurance commissioner John Oxendine had been running and raising money for some time. Lieutenant Governor Casey Cagle had announced his candidacy in late 2008. Neither had the broad backing from the GOP. Alternatives were being floated. I was one.

I formally announced my candidacy for governor that April.

It would be a crowded, changing field. Oxendine was in for the long haul. Cagle dropped out early and ran for reelection as lieutenant governor. This prompted Eric Johnson, then President Pro Tem of the Georgia Senate, to drop his bid for lieutenant governor and set his sights on the governorship. Then, Congressman Nathan Deal jumped in.[2] Current congressman Austin Scott was originally running for governor before jumping into the congressional race and eventually defeating incumbent Jim Marshall. States' rights advocate Ray McBerry and state senator Jeff Chapman also joined the fray.

My decision was cheered—and criticized. Many were enthusiastic about my reform-minded, no-nonsense approach. Others said I was overly ambitious—my rise up the political ladder was too quick. I was only forty-nine, so what was the rush? Interestingly, these criticisms had not been raised about the lieutenant governor, who is four years younger than I, when he decided to run just two years into his first term. And while it was fine for a woman to be secretary of state, a woman running for governor raised eyebrows.

Contrary to news reports during the week of Komen's short-lived split from Planned Parenthood, my campaign was not based on an "aggressive anti-abortion and anti–Planned Parenthood" platform. Rather, jobs, the economy, reforming the tax code and state government, and ethics reform were the key issues. I had a strong record of success on each. I had more private sector experience than any of the other announced candidates. I was a fresh face—relatively new to elected office in comparison to the others. Georgia seemed ready for someone like me with my business experience. I knew it would be tough, but I also knew I was the right person at the right time for my state—a state that had given me so much.

———

Fund-raising was difficult—again. It was even more difficult this time around, because as secretary of state I was prohibited from accepting corporate contributions from any entity that held a professional license in the state, putting me at a significant financial disadvantage. Every other week, we had to fend off rumors that I was dropping out. I was not moving in the polls.

By December, my campaign leadership had reached the conclusion that, if I wanted a chance at being governor, I would have to resign as secretary of state.

I resisted vehemently. I had been elected to serve a four-year term. I took this responsibility seriously and was not going to let down the people who put their confidence in me. I would be called a quitter. I was angry that I had to run under a different set of rules than my opponents. I was angry at being pushed into a corner, with two ways out, both undesirable: remain as secretary of state and put the campaign in jeopardy; or resign, which I believed would disappoint those who had supported me.

Being secretary of state was a full-time job with full-time responsibilities and a full-time salary. Georgians had a right to expect my full-time devotion. On the other hand, a campaign for governor was also a full-time endeavor, and those supporting me had a right to expect my complete commitment.

On December 30, 2009, I resigned as secretary of state—to run for governor full-time.

━━━━

We knew we needed to make a move soon to gain some traction. Ethics was my opening to shake things up. Unlike my opponents, I did not have baggage in the ethics department. I had to go for it. And I did.

On January 5, 2010, before a crowd of nearly four hundred women, I made the culture of the capitol a key issue. I laid out my plan for ethics reform—a gift ban, real conflict of interest restrictions, a cooling-off period before legislators could turn to lobbying, a fully funded ethics commission with teeth and the ability to actually enforce the rules, and the same open-records requirements for the legislature that applied to the rest of state government. And I did it with a bang.

I was introduced by Rear Admiral Marty Evans (retired), the highest-ranking female officer in the United States Navy, who, ironically, had led the investigation into the Tailhook scandal twenty years earlier.

The speech was titled "Sex, Lies, and Lobbyists."

It would be the turning point in the campaign.

"It is time for leadership that will shake things up and clean things up."

"I'm not saying that only a woman can do this . . . what I am saying is that this woman—as your next governor—can and will."

My poll numbers jumped. We knew all along I had a shot, but now others were starting to believe it, too.

But it was a turning point in another sense as well.

Most of the legislators were unhappy—irate. I dared to shine a light on their club and had the audacity to say what most people were already thinking—and continue to think even today. While I had a few legislators in my camp, most were aligned with one of the other candidates—a fellow member of the good-old-boys club.

We knew that making ethics front and center of the campaign would be controversial. We also knew that ethics was a real difference between my opponents and me. But for me ethics was something bigger and more important than a campaign talking point. I would recall Mike Bowers' words from my first months in public office—what kind of an elected official will you be? One who sees a problem and ignores it? Or one who sees a problem and works to fix it? Our system was broken, and I was determined to do something about it. One only has to look at the remarkable transformation in Louisiana under Governor Bobby Jindal or New Jersey under Governor Chris Christie to see what truly transformational conservatives can do for citizens.

John Oxendine was already under investigation for allegedly taking $100,000 in excess, illegal campaign contributions.[3]

Ray McBerry had his teaching certificate suspended because of an inappropriate relationship with a sixteen-year-old student he was counseling.[4] When he continued to be invited to GOP debates, I called on the party to distance itself from McBerry and refused to be on the same stage with him.

As a woman, I was repulsed. But I was stunned that not one of my opponents—all fellow Republicans, supposed conservatives, and importantly, fathers—shared my disgust. Instead they joined McBerry in criticizing me for raising the issue at all.

State senator Eric Johnson failed to investigate allegations of misconduct against the Republican Speaker, allegations that would later be proven true.[5] He also failed to properly disclose $200,000 in state contracts with his architecture firm.[6]

Nathan Deal had been named one of the most corrupt politicians in Washington. The nonpartisan Office of Congressional

Ethics (OCE) found Deal had taken "active steps" to protect a state contract that netted his company nearly $300,000 a year, while also exceeding the limits set on outside income for members of Congress.[7] The report recommended further investigation, and the matter was referred to the congressional ethics committee. On March 21 at 11:45 p.m., Deal resigned—just one day before the ethics committee's deadline to act.[8] The resignation allowed him to campaign full-time for governor and escape the jurisdiction of the congressional committee.[9]

Later, still more alleged serious ethical lapses would come to light.

Deal failed to report millions of dollars in business loans on his federal financial disclosures and his personal financial disclosures filed to run for governor.[10]

Then he was accused of illegally using funds from his governor's campaign account to pay for lawyers to defend him against the congressional ethics charges. And there was more. An investigative report by the *Atlanta Journal-Constitution* revealed that Deal was benefiting personally through a complex arrangement involving a plane leased from a Deal-owned company by the Deal campaign.[11]

However, I would soon learn that, despite these ethical questions, Georgia GOP primaries eventually came down to who was the most conservative—specifically, who was the *most* pro-life.

I would have my next run-in with Georgia Right to Life and my first real encounter with bullies on the abortion issue—and it would come from the right, not the pro-choice left.

Georgia Right to Life

I entered my meeting with GRTL with my typical Pollyanna enthusiasm. My pro-life views were the same. There should be no surprises for anyone. While I still supported exceptions in the case of rape and incest, I really thought that this time I would make my case. Surely the opportunity to have a woman as governor, a woman who was deeply pro-life, would be viewed positively, as an opportunity for the cause. Yes, we still had areas of disagreements, but we agreed on far more.

Dan Becker, GRTL's president, led the meeting.

The discussion seemed to be going well. Then fertility treatments were mentioned.

I was immediately uncomfortable, and my focus drifted as the sadness and pain of not having a child pushed their way to the surface. Then I thought I heard Becker say something about fertility treatments being immoral, that they would be outlawed.

I stopped. What did he just say? Obviously, I had misheard or misunderstood. What do fertility treatments have to do with pro-abortion or pro-life?

During our nearly ten-year journey, Steve and I tried nearly every fertility treatment that was available at the time—all to no avail. We considered in vitro but opted against it, only because our doctor advised that the chances of a successful pregnancy would not be improved with the procedure. But if a married couple can benefit from fertility treatments, including in vitro, who was I to prevent that couple from being a family—to prevent that woman from being a mom? With that kind of stance, how could I honestly face married couples—like the many we knew—who had become parents with the help of fertility procedures? Was Becker saying that I would have to denounce these parents as immoral?

Our meeting lasted more than two hours. I pushed Becker to explain. He went off on a tangent about the California "Octomom"—as if this single mother who already had six other children and was having eight more through in vitro was a fair representation of the hundreds of thousands of married couples pursuing fertility in hopes of having even just one child of their own.

Finally, frustrated, I asked. "Dan, do you have children?" I can still recall the exchange as if it occurred yesterday.

Becker said, "Yes, several."

I could feel the condescension in his reply but maintained my control and simply said, "You're very blessed. Were you able to have them without any assistance?"

"Of course!" he replied.

"Well, then," I said, "you're extraordinarily blessed. Perhaps this explains your lack of empathy or compassion for a husband and a wife who are simply trying to have a family like you."

Becker came across as callous and insensitive, revealing a sense of arrogance that those who can have children (on their own) are somehow better—superior—than those who cannot.

The meeting was over. I would not get the endorsement, and we all understood that the impact in the governor's race would be far greater than in the secretary of state's race. If this meant losing the race, I would accept that. But I was not—am not—prepared to tell a husband and wife that they are evil and immoral if they have the miracle of a child through fertility treatments.

GRTL Picks a Fight

On June 3, GRTL issued its endorsements, but this time they took a decidedly different approach than in the past. GRTL frequently did not endorse candidates, but its focus had always been on those being endorsed, saying virtually nothing about those who were not. But not this time. This time GRTL dedicated the majority of the ink in its announcement for the one candidate it was not supporting: me.[12]

The *Atlanta Journal-Constitution* column was headlined GRTL PICKS FIGHT WITH HANDEL. GRTL said I didn't meet the "21st Century demands of being pro-life," that I supported "abortion based on the manner of conception," and that I did not believe an embryo was a "human child." Becker knew this to be untrue but needed stark, dark imagery to justify the attack. The fertility rationale was a tenuous one for GRTL. In 2009, the legislature, with GRTL's backing, had tried to ban most fertility treatments, and the public backlash was fierce.

We pushed back. If GRTL wanted a fight, I would give them one. All the while, though, I was wondering just why GRTL had decided that I had to be singled out and attacked.

Not content to let the issue go, Becker issued a second statement. This time he crossed every line of common decency, saying that Steve and I—and other husbands and wives like us—were "desperate" and "barren."[13]

The silence from my opponents and other Republican leaders was deafening and, I am not embarrassed to admit, hurtful. Even the Democrats were silent—relishing the idea that I was taking a huge hit, and knowing that if one of the others was the nominee, his silence in this moment could be a rallying cry for women.

All I could see was the hypocrisy of it all.

The other candidates had simply checked the right boxes—followed the staff-written talking points—afraid of any repercussions that challenging GRTL would bring. They'd never be called on to explain their positions. They'd never be asked to think through real-life consequences of their daughter being raped and becoming pregnant as a result. They had not gone through the pain of infertility—or at least, none admitted to it.

Deal received GRTL's endorsement despite various pro-choice votes during his tenure in the U.S. House of Representatives. Ironically, Deal and Becker were once opponents, facing off in the 1992 congressional race. Deal was still a Democrat then, and Becker, the Republican, had based his entire campaign on Deal's pro-abortion votes and views. Apparently, by checking all of the boxes, all was forgiven.

GRTL even endorsed McBerry. He, too, apparently checked the boxes.

My opponents were gleeful, and rightly so—this was a huge break for them.

A few weeks later, when asked if she thought I was pro-life, Georgia Republican Party chairman Sue Everhart answered unequivocally, "yes."

My opponents cried foul, accusing Everhart of giving me "cover." As chairman, she should not be engaged at all, they argued.[14] I was grateful that finally at least one Republican leader was willing to stand up to the GRTL bullies.

Just eight days before the primary, a "game changer" occurred in the race—or at least, that's what the press called it. Former GOP vice presidential nominee Sarah Palin endorsed my candidacy.

GRTL reacted immediately, offering this: "[Palin] has a son with Down's Syndrome, and under Karen Handel's laws, Handel would have felt like it was ok to go in and abort that child," GRTL executive director Melanie Crozier told *Politico*. "But when you look at Sarah Palin's pattern—going out finding mainly women candidates that were in the lead and endorsing them, that's not really a surprise. She saw Handel had a decent lead, so I think she sort of jumped on the bandwagon."[15]

I could not believe what Crozier had said. My sister had been born with a serious, life-threatening congenital condition. Was she actually saying that I would have been okay with my sister being aborted? GRTL had stepped over the line once more. All I could think of was how my sister would feel.

Once again, my opponents were silent, chiming in only to slam Governor Palin's endorsement. The head of the Georgia 9-12 Project, also a Deal supporter, offered, "Georgians don't endorse candidates because they wear lipstick." Johnson's campaign noted their surprise that Palin had endorsed the "most liberal Republican in the race." And from the Deal camp: it's disappointing that "Palin has chosen to back the most liberal Republican in the race." The blogs were filled with rants about the endorsement being nothing more than one woman supporting another.[16]

Palin's endorsement was a lift to my campaign and would later be used to boost the left's portrait of me as an anti-abortion radical.

On July 20, I was the top vote-getter in the primary, with 34 percent. Deal finished second, with 23 percent. We would face each other in the August 10 runoff.

Runoffs and Abortion

The runoff was just twenty days away—August 10. And the Gold Dome clique was nervous. I was continuing to talk about ethics reform—promising an end to their way of doing things. They rallied around Nathan Deal.

At the same time, I was being hammered on the abortion issue, and I was being called pro-gay. I had spoken to the gay Republican group Log Cabin Republicans and had sponsored one of their events during an earlier campaign for the Fulton County commission.

Deal had his opening to question my conservative values.

In the first days of the runoff, we hit Deal hard with a scorching mail piece highlighting dozens of press headlines from the extensive coverage of his ethics issues. Deal cried foul, working to make the case that I was negative and not talking about the issues. In our next debate, I pointed out that his ethics issues *were* issues. How could we trust a governor to run the state's finances when he couldn't run his own? In a debate, I said that campaigns were tough and perhaps Deal needed to "put his big boy pants on."

Polls continued to have me in the lead. We were cautiously optimistic. Meanwhile, Deal seemed to be drawing on every connection he'd ever had in Congress and calling in every marker. Deal's campaign took in more than $130,000 of over-the-legal-limit campaign contributions, a matter that as of today remains under investigation.[17]

Word was circulating that former Arkansas governor Mike Huckabee might engage in the race somehow. We knew Huckabee was close to Deal, but we had our ties to Huckabee, too. My campaign manager Marty Ryall, who is from Arkansas, knew Huckabee well and gave him a call. Huckabee said he was staying out of the race. Neutral was just fine with us.

Then, without any heads-up, despite his long friendship with Marty, Huckabee endorsed . . . Deal.[18]

We were caught off guard. Not so much from the endorsement itself, but because Huckabee's endorsement brought a fresh round of attacks from the pro-life right. Flyers were placed on cars at the large churches around Georgia, spewing an array of outrageous lies—and all anonymously.

I lost. Deal won, with 50.2 percent of the vote to my 49.8 percent. A margin of victory of just 2,519 votes of 579,551 votes cast—less than one vote per precinct.

Facing Defeat

It was a devastating loss. My supporters wanted a recount. I was legally entitled to it but decided against it. I was the former secretary of state and, though the race was very close, the likelihood that a recount would change the overall outcome was slim. We had a great team. Our strategy was on target. We worked hard, executed well. We just came up a little short. Being gracious in defeat—no matter how hard—was what I expected of myself and what I knew my supporters expected of me, too.

I called Deal the following morning and conceded. He expressed his surprise and was anything but gracious in victory.

I'm often asked what I would have done differently in the campaign. Would I have pushed ethics less? No. Would I have caved to Georgia Right to Life and simply checked the right boxes? Absolutely not, even though the abortion issue gave Deal—the former pro-abortion Democrat with significant ethics issues—the victory.

Today, the irony of this is not lost on me. Little did I know that I would soon be the poster child for irony—trying to reconcile GRTL's attacks against me for not being pro-life enough with the Planned Parenthood bullies who vilified me as a pro-life zealot.

2

From the Frying Pan

After the election, I took a much-needed break. Deal's camp was not interested in my help, and the truth was, I needed a vacation. Steve and I packed up Maggie and Mia, our Cavalier King Charles spaniels, and headed to the beach. After a few days, Steve returned to Atlanta. After about two weeks, I readied myself to face whatever was next, figuring I'd better get home before I acted on my sudden urge to set up shop renting bicycles on the side of the road.

I was already bored. Sitting around, focusing on what wasn't—that wasn't for me. The general election was still more than two months off, so it was too early to put my resume on the street. Besides, I hadn't sorted out what was next. But I needed something to do—a challenge for myself. That challenge was running—literally. I'd never run before (except campaigns, of course). My goal: 5K by Christmas. I did it—and in the process, got in better shape and used the time to reflect and rejuvenate. Today I'm an avid runner, covering twelve to fifteen miles of pavement a week.

In December, I formed the Handel Strategy Group and began talking with friends and contacts about consulting opportunities.

I got a call from my old friend Rae. She had once again been invaluable in helping me look ahead with optimism, and she had an idea. "The Komen folks can really use your help," she said, based on her work with them over the past twenty years.

I'd had some experience with Susan G. Komen for the Cure, during my time with Marilyn Quayle. I knew Nancy Brinker, the founder and CEO of Komen, but I hadn't seen her in years, except for a brief exchange at the 2008 Republican National Convention in Minneapolis. I'm certain she did not remember me.

I had stayed somewhat involved with breast cancer awareness issues over the year, and as an elected official, I was always willing to participate in breast-cancer-related activities, although it was mostly through the American Cancer Society. So the idea of reengaging on the issue was very appealing. Komen had a good reputation. Ending breast cancer was something everyone could rally around. No controversies. No uproars. And it was about as far away as I could get from the abortion/pro-life debate.

I met with several members of Komen's management, including its president, Liz Thompson. She filled me in.

States across the country were facing significant budget gaps. Komen feared cuts in state matching funds for the National Breast and Cervical Cancer Early Detection Program (NBCCEDP). NBCCEDP is a federal program, run by the Centers for Disease Control and Prevention, that provides matching funds to states for mammograms to uninsured and underinsured women who are not eligible for Medicaid. The program is administered directly by government agencies in some states, and in other states through contracts to outside organizations—including Planned Parenthood, I would later learn. Komen received none of this funding. In fact, except for a few instances in which Komen receives revenue from breast cancer license plates, the organization receives no government funding.

Komen was concerned that it lacked the expertise to be effective in preserving the funds for this program. The intricacies of the state budget process were little understood. Komen also found itself lacking in key state capital relationships following the 2010 elections, which was a "red tide" that swept in enough Republicans to give the GOP the majority of governors and flip twenty state legislatures from Democrat to Republican majorities.

This was right up my alley. I knew state budgets. I understood the legislative process. I had contacts across the country with governors and legislative leadership. I was a Republican—which was exactly what Komen wanted. Later, much would be made about my political affiliation, and questions would be raised about the prudence of hiring someone with a political background for the public policy role. This was a red herring. I was not hired because of my personal ideology. I was hired because of my abilities and, yes, my political contacts. In the world of public policy, that's how it works. If 2010 had been a "blue surge" that established new Democratic majorities, Komen would have been looking for someone from the other side of the aisle. And rightly so.

Preserving the funding would be no easy task, I advised. The states were under severe financial constraints. No program—no matter how worthwhile—would be exempt from scrutiny and possible cuts. Our issue was one that most people would be sympathetic toward, but we would still have some real fights ahead of us. I remember one Komen executive wondering aloud if "Komen had the stomach for it." These words seemed innocuous at that time. Months later, I would recall them as an ominous foreshadowing.

I was hired. My first gig as a consultant. Life was moving forward.

Within weeks, Liz asked me to "manage" the public policy team. This was an unusual request of a consultant. I learned that there had been several policy vice presidents in just a few years and no manager in months. The team was in flux—which was making my work more difficult. I agreed to do it.

Very soon after, Nancy and Liz began asking me to consider the senior vice president role. I resisted.

In March, I caught my first glimpse of Komen's liberal leanings. There's no politics in breast cancer, I thought. We had brought together a group of Komen local affiliate leaders who had been involved in state policy issues, along with the entire Komen National policy team. I met a wall of hostility and open anger toward Republicans. One affiliate leader actually called a governor "just another Republican Neanderthal." Another, in response to an idea, commented that we had better not do that because the new Republican governor would "have you arrested."

Nancy and Liz continued to press for me to join Komen full-time. I knew it would be a challenging role. Komen had some turnover issues, especially among management, and the animosity toward Republicans was a bit disconcerting. But I was undaunted. I loved challenges—I was a good worker, a professional; I would be successful. Plus, the idea of a stable job—rather than consulting—was appealing. I was a problem solver; Komen had problems. I knew I could make a positive contribution.

My appointment was announced with great fanfare by Nancy at the annual Komen Leadership Conference before nearly one thousand Komen affiliate executive directors, board members, and staff. Liz was thrilled, Nancy ecstatic. The policy team and others greeted the news with open hostility.

I started on April 4, 2011.

The Players

Komen was politically and personally eclectic—and pink was everywhere.

Ambassador Nancy Brinker is the founder and current CEO of Komen. She is driven, passionate, visionary.

Nancy is also a Republican and has had appointments in every Republican administration since Reagan. Because of her Republican ties, many assumed that Komen itself is a right-leaning organization; that Nancy built a far-right culture. They are wrong.

To a great degree, Nancy is Komen. But the culture within the organization had little to do with her and nothing to do with her politics. Nancy did not take on the role of CEO until November 2009. Prior to that, dating back to at least 1996, others held the post of president/CEO, while Nancy sat on the board, serving as the face of the organization. For most of the past decade, because of her political appointments, Nancy had to distance herself from any formal role. From 2001 to 2003, she was the ambassador to Hungary. From 2007 to January 2009, she was chief of protocol at the U.S. State Department.

Nancy has solid Republican credibility, but she is hardly the card-carrying, hard-core conservative the media and liberals have made her out to be. Several people have mentioned to me that Nancy once wanted to run for U.S. Senate in Florida, but conservatives rejected that notion—she was not pro-life. In the 1990s, she served on the board of the Dallas chapter of Planned Parenthood and was even given the group's humanitarian award. In August 2011, President Obama awarded her the Presidential Medal of Freedom, calling her "a catalyst to ease suffering in the world."

Nancy is a dynamic, inspirational leader. We did not always agree, but I offered my opinion candidly, and to her credit, she always heard me out. She was the CEO and free to take my counsel or leave it. She didn't hire me to be her rubber stamp.

She could also be very vulnerable to criticism, especially in the press. As I would find out, this was an influential factor in a time of crisis.

Komen's president was Elizabeth Thompson, who had been president since September 2010, a few months before I arrived. Before that, she'd been the senior vice president of medical and scientific affairs, managing the research portfolio and overseeing the community grants program.

Liz is extremely knowledgeable about the science of breast

cancer—early detection, treatment, and research—and about community granting. Her passion for the mission is unmistakable, and she has a rare ability to truly connect with the women we served—especially those who called seeking her counsel after just being diagnosed.

However, when it came to being president—to leading the organization—she sometimes seemed a bit out of her depth. I expected Komen's president to be a seasoned professional who was decisive and commanding. At times Liz seemed unsure, unwilling to make the tough calls, and easily backed off a position, especially if there was not unanimity.

Liz and I quickly developed a very positive rapport. I did my job well, and she and Nancy took notice, happy to have someone managing the group in D.C. and delivering wins for our advocacy efforts on the state budgets and preserving funding for the breast cancer screening programs across the country.

Liz and Cecile Richards, head of Planned Parenthood, were friends. They frequently crossed paths and had sat on numerous panels together. That would come into play later.

Mollie Williams was the managing director of community health, overseeing Komen's nearly $100 million community grant portfolio. Developing Komen's overall grants strategy and setting the guidelines under which Komen affiliates made their local grants fell under Mollie's jurisdiction. Mollie was a major proponent of Planned Parenthood. Her Twitter and Facebook were littered with gushing declarations about Planned Parenthood. She had volunteered at Planned Parenthood of Austin when she attended the University of Texas.

Mollie was unreceptive toward me from my first days at Komen. Although we never discussed it, I always sensed that my personal political views were the reason.

Mollie was my main point of contact regarding the details of Komen's overall grants process, and specifically on Planned Parenthood grants. She was not always as cooperative as I would have liked and getting information from her could be tedious and time-consuming—and usually required Liz to weigh in. While I had hoped to work productively with Mollie, I was disappointed when that was not the case.

One of Mollie's close friends was John Hammarley, a press person in Komen's communications department until a reorganization affected his position. One of the first emails I received about Planned Parenthood after joining Komen originated with John. It contained derogatory comments about pro-lifers, prompting me to respond to Nancy and Liz that the statements seemed inappropriate and that our focus was our mission. I don't think I ever met John or discussed the Planned Parenthood situation with him directly, but John would later position himself with the media as having direct, inside information on the situation and my involvement.

Leslie Aun was Komen's vice president of communications, and we both worked out of Komen's D.C. office. She joined the organization at about the same time as I did, working under Katrina McGhee, the executive vice president of marketing. Leslie had an impressive communications background. She had previously held senior communications positions with the liberal environmental groups World Wildlife Fund and Earth Hour, as well as with the Special Olympics. She was also an adjunct professor of communications at Georgetown University.

I assumed that most at Komen knew my personal political views, but I rarely talked about those views at the office. Leslie seemed to want to ensure that everyone knew her politics. Shortly after I joined Komen, I learned that Leslie regularly referred to me as "the righty tighty"—whatever that means. To her credit, Leslie came to me and apologized. Over the next few months, we became friends—or so I thought.

Leslie seemed to be struggling to gain her footing within Komen. Outside consultants were relied on more and more. Eventually, Nancy asked Republican strategist Ari Fleischer to lead a search for a senior communications person.[1]

Leslie's boss was Katrina McGhee. As executive vice president of marketing, Katrina was responsible for revenue generation, including cause-related marketing, corporate and foundation giving, the Global Race for the Cure, the 3-Day race, and online fund-raising. She was also a key liaison with Komen's corporate donor leadership, alongside Liz and Nancy.

I was probably like most people when they first meet Katrina—I was wowed. She is very sharp, with a keen marketing mind. But as I got to know her, to see her in action, her wow factor faded and my respect for her waned. She, too, seemed to lack the kind of leadership and management skills that one would expect in such a senior role. I suspected that there were those who feared Katrina more than respected her. But Katrina brought in the money, so that earned her a pass.

Nancy, Liz, Katrina, and I, along with Komen's general

counsel, CFO, and several other top executives, were Komen's Operating Committee.

Komen's Board of Directors was composed of savvy, influential leaders. It was diverse in gender, race—and politics.

Komen is an "affiliated network" of more than 120 local autonomous Komen organizations. Each affiliate has its own executive director and board. The affiliates manage the local Races for the Cure and are Komen's community leaders, distributing more than $93 million a year in grants to nearly two thousand nonprofits. The affiliates have varying degrees of experience—some are very large with highly skilled staff, while others are very small and staffed by volunteers. The relationship between the Affiliate Network and Komen National, headquartered in Dallas, Texas, was sometimes strained—much like relationships between corporate headquarters and field offices can be.

My first months at Komen were spent reorganizing the policy team and focusing on the state budget initiative. As I worked with the affiliates and became more familiar with Komen and my colleagues, it became apparent to me that the organization and most of those with whom I worked were more liberal in their thinking. Komen had not endorsed President Obama's healthcare reform bill, instead issuing a more middle-of-the-road "statement of principles." This seemed to be a bone of contention for many within Komen. I experienced open disdain for Republicans on a regular basis. There was little understanding of the realities of how policy and legislation were advanced. In most states, there were new majorities, many Republican. I underscored the importance of Komen maintaining positive relationships on *both* sides of the aisle. Eventually the affiliates and the policy team itself established a partnership—more of convenience than congeniality. Together we were successful in preserving the funding for the breast screening program in virtually every state.

Nancy and Liz were by all accounts quite pleased with my performance and the new energy and focus of the team. On my ninety-day anniversary with Komen, Liz sent me a glowing note and a spa gift certificate. Things were good. After the partisan insanity of Georgia politics, working at Komen was a relief.

Introducing Planned Parenthood

In 1916, Margaret Sanger founded a local birth control clinic in Brooklyn, New York. It was the first clinic of its type in the country and would serve as the foundation of today's Planned Parenthood. In 1923, Sanger opened the Birth Control Clinic Research Bureau in Manhattan and also established the American Birth Control League. Eventually, the two organizations merged and Planned Parenthood Federation of America was born. While Sanger was said to have been an active proponent of eugenics (the sterilization or abortion of certain populations), rumors that she supported forced sterilization and targeted abortion based on race are untrue. She did, however, pursue sterilization of the severely mentally disabled.

Over the years, Planned Parenthood grew into an enormously successful organization with an annual budget of more than $1 billion. This budget, however, is boosted by hundreds of millions of dollars in federal, state, and local government funding.

The vast majority of Planned Parenthood activities—97 percent—are not related to abortion, at least according to Planned Parenthood. Outside studies are more revealing. Planned Parenthood distorts its numbers through the way it defines a "service." In calculating its claim that 97 percent of its services are not abortion-related, Planned Parenthood counts the distribution of a single condom as a service, just like an abortion is counted as a service.[2]

Whatever the reality, Planned Parenthood *is* the country's leading abortion provider. In 2010, Planned Parenthood performed 329,445 surgical abortions or abortions using the RU486 pill, commonly known as the morning-after pill, which is generally used for abortions up to nine weeks into a pregnancy, according to Planned Parenthood.[3] That's more than 27 percent of all abortions performed in the United States every year. While Planned Parenthood emphasizes that the vast majority of its services are not abortions, a closer look at the number of other services provided offers a different perspective. In 2010, just over 30,000 prenatal "services" were provided—that's the equivalent of 5,398 women receiving these services. Further, just 841 adoption referrals were made.[4]

Abortion, like government funding, is big money for Planned Parenthood. According to an analysis of Planned Parenthood's 2010 annual report by watchdog group Stop Planned Parenthood, abortion income accounted for approximately 51.5 percent of all of Planned Parenthood's nongovernment income.[5]

So how does Komen fit into all of this? Sixteen percent of Planned Parenthood's budget is dedicated to cancer screening and prevention.[6] Planned Parenthood had been receiving grants from Komen affiliates for two decades or perhaps longer, and the relationship between the two organizations ran deep—at the national level and among the Komen affiliate leadership. Nancy had even once served on the board of the Dallas Planned Parenthood chapter. Both she and Liz had participated in numerous events and panels with Cecile Richards and others from Planned Parenthood. At the local level, Komen affiliates and Planned Parenthood chapters walked in the same circles, and some Komen affiliate board members had previously served on Planned Parenthood local boards, and vice versa.

But, as Nancy and Liz remarked frequently, the mission of Planned Parenthood had changed over time, and so had its role in the community and in politics. When Komen first began the grants, Planned Parenthood was one of the only resources in low-income communities. But since then the infrastructure and number of programs to serve low-resource women have expanded. While Planned Parenthood conducted education and outreach programs, Planned Parenthood had never provided mammograms, and still doesn't. It provides referrals or, as is the case today with a few chapters, contracts with another organization for mobile mammography services—a new approach in an attempt to bolster its claims as a breast health provider.

As time went on, Planned Parenthood's emphasis on and forceful public advocacy for abortion fueled significant controversy. Then, when Cecile Richards took the reins as president, Planned Parenthood began to engage aggressively in partisan politics, establishing scores of political action committees—

nationally and in the states—to provide a platform from which to elect pro–Planned Parenthood officials. Together, these issues made Komen an increasing target, causing some to question the relationship and creating concerns within Komen.

"Crappy Grants"

One of Liz's top priorities was implementing what is called an "outcomes-based" granting strategy. Komen would employ a methodical approach to achieving measurable outcomes in the fight against breast cancer. Liz spoke with great passion and excitement about the initiative, and I got the sense that this was the legacy she wanted to leave from her tenure as president.

Komen could not afford to continue granting in the same old way. Dollars were harder and harder to come by. Donors expected that their contributions actually made a difference— that there be a real, tangible impact—in the fight against breast cancer. Komen's board was also demanding measurable outcomes. Komen was no longer the fledgling nonprofit—it was a global leader, and that came with greater expectations and higher responsibilities.

Through its local affiliates, Komen had a considerable community granting portfolio, investing more than $93 million in community grants for breast health education, awareness, and screening services with nearly two thousand nonprofits. Komen invests millions more in scientific research into breast cancer causes, detection, prevention, and treatment.

There was a deep understanding that higher standards—

for the programs and the organizations administering those programs—were required. We could quantify our success in terms of the number of people we served, but we lacked a systematic way to evaluate our grants and measure their true impact. With a more methodical approach and defined metrics, Komen would be able to track shifts in attitudes and behaviors. We would be able to measure actual improvements in health outcomes. Were our efforts improving survival rates? Were we lowering the number of deaths from breast cancer through our programs?

Under this new approach, vague goals, such as "raising awareness" or "educating women," would no longer be enough. Funding the creation and distribution of education materials would also not meet these new standards. We would strive to be more cost-effective and efficient by moving away from what is called pass-through grants—whereby dollars are granted to one organization that then contracts with another entity to actually provide the service.

Many long-standing Komen grants, including the vast majority of Planned Parenthood's grants, would not meet the goals of this new granting model and would be unable to live up to these higher standards and more stringent requirements.

"Crappy grants"—that's how Liz referred to the Planned Parenthood grants. I don't believe she was in any way implying that Planned Parenthood was doing a crappy job or that it was a crappy organization. Rather, I think she was simply saying that these grants would not meet the higher standards that we would be demanding going forward.

I was surprised by this characterization of Planned Parenthood grants—and others like them. As I learned more about the actual Planned Parenthood initiatives that Komen funded, I gained an appreciation for what we were trying to do by evolving the grants strategy. It made perfect sense: get the biggest bang for each dollar invested. Further, if the Planned Parenthood grants were not delivering the kind of results we wanted, it made little sense for us to continue absorbing PR hits and alienating a significant pool of potential donors. These grants were not essential to Komen's overall efforts, and it would become apparent that these dollars were also not essential to Planned Parenthood or its mission, either.

In fiscal year 2010 (April 1–March 31), nineteen Komen affiliates awarded grants totaling approximately $600,000 to Planned Parenthood. Planned Parenthood chapters received approximately $700,000 from sixteen Komen Affiliates in fiscal year 2011. (Note: The dollar amounts of the grants vary from those reported in the media because the two organizations operate on different financial calendars.) The majority of these were repeat grants, funded some years in a row.

Many of the grants funded education programs or education materials. Educating women about breast cancer is obviously important, but the underlying goal isn't just getting women to attend a seminar. The real goal is for women to actually follow through with their annual mammograms and achieve improved health outcomes.

A number of the grants combined education with "free" clinical breast exams (CBE), a physical examination of a woman's breast by a health-care professional. A CBE is considered a standard part of any well-woman checkup, and as Planned Parenthood notes in a video on its website, CBE is part of most annual gynecological exams it offers.[7] The American College of Obstetricians & Gynecologists, the American Cancer Society, and Komen all recommend that a CBE be included in a woman's annual checkup. Moreover, CBE is specifically covered under Medicare; most state Medicaid programs and private insurance also cover CBE.[8]

These grants raised a couple of questions.

First, Komen's grant dollars cannot be used for services that are reimbursable by insurance or other programs, such as Medicare and Medicaid. How did Planned Parenthood ensure that it met this requirement? Did they have a tracking process to allocate grant dollars only to those who qualified?

Second, in most instances, education and CBEs were grouped together. How much went to education and how much for CBEs? How many women were really receiving direct breast health services that were unique to Komen's grant versus something that Planned Parenthood would have provided anyway?

Third, would Planned Parenthood actually stop providing CBEs during its well-woman checkup without the grant? That seemed unlikely—if not highly unethical—especially since there was no added cost involved.

A number of the Planned Parenthood grants went to programs to educate women about monthly breast self-examination, or BSE. For years, Komen advocated BSE as an early detection method; but in recent years, after science began to question the effectiveness, Komen stopped recommending it.

My question: Why was Planned Parenthood still receiving

grants to educate women about the importance of something that was no longer recommended?

Planned Parenthood especially liked to promote itself as a provider of mammograms to poor women. The truth is, Planned Parenthood does *not* provide mammograms. Planned Parenthood *refers* women to mammography providers, serving as the middlewoman, if you will. But Planned Parenthood even overstated this. In fiscal year 2010, just four of the nineteen grants actually provided any dollars to pay for mammograms—again, through referrals. This was roughly $100,000 of the total amount in grants. If a woman received a referral, did she actually follow through in obtaining the mammogram? How did Planned Parenthood know who actually obtained a mammogram and who didn't?

In some of the grants, Planned Parenthood made promises that simply could not be kept—or at least, there was no way to really know. For example, a Planned Parenthood chapter in New Jersey received just over $43,000. Here's what they said they would "achieve" with these dollars: increase the number of patients and education program participants who receive mammograms; ensure appropriate services if an abnormality is detected during a clinical breast exam; educate 800 women age 40 or older; provide 550 clinical breast exams to women over 40; and navigate approximately 80 patients through the health-care system. When I read this, I thought, wow, this grant does a lot—and all for less than fifty thousand dollars! But when I looked closer, the cracks appeared.

Planned Parenthood had no way to know if, in fact, they

were increasing the number of women receiving mammograms. They weren't providing mammograms. Planned Parenthood also said that the grant dollars would be used to make referrals if an abnormality were found. Surely Planned Parenthood does this anyway—with or without a grant from Komen or anyone else.

───

The more I learned about the Planned Parenthood grants, the more I understood exactly why Komen had to change its granting strategy. One grant claimed it would save 450 women from dying of breast cancer. That is an amazing claim and one that we all wish were true. Of course, there was no way for Planned Parenthood to guarantee this as an outcome to its program.

Another Planned Parenthood chapter received grants for at least two consecutive years to fund breast evaluation and management of low-risk women between the ages of 18 and 39 in order to avoid unnecessary treatment and to minimize the burden on the health-care system from the so-called worried well. This grant was particularly odd to me and had the smell of flowery application wording, focused more on keeping the dollars flowing than on actually addressing a real need.

In addition to improving the quality and outcomes of our grants, Komen was pursuing stronger oversight of its grants and grantees. With more than $93 million in community grants each year, we had a responsibility to ensure that these grant dollars were being used appropriately, effectively, and in accordance with our goals and the grant contract.

My questions about grant accountability led to one of my

most unpleasant encounters with Mollie. Our press statements about Planned Parenthood said that twice-yearly audits were conducted. I was shocked to learn that there were no audits. Grantees provided twice-yearly reports and periodic site visits were conducted, but there were no actual audits. After my experiences at the Chamber of Commerce and in government, I have learned that self-reporting is fine only up to a point. When other people's money is at stake, robust accountability and audits are needed.

I asked specifically about the mammogram referrals. Many women, even those with insurance coverage, receive a referral yet unfortunately never follow through with actually getting their mammogram. The same would be true with women receiving a referral from Planned Parenthood. How did Planned Parenthood actually track this and report it? It seemed highly unlikely that every referral resulted in a mammogram that Planned Parenthood paid for out of the Komen grant dollars. Did Planned Parenthood provide documentation to confirm the payments? If funds went unused, were they returned? Mollie seemed angry and offended by my questions, noting pointedly that trust between Komen and its grantees was imperative.

I understood that trust was important. But so was accountability. As Ronald Reagan said: Trust, but verify.

With the intense backlash over the years, Komen did its best to put the most positive spin on the Planned Parenthood grants, emphasizing that the funds to Planned Parenthood were a very,

very small percentage of Komen's overall granting portfolio. However, some of the statements in the materials were outdated.

"In many cases," read one press statement, "Planned Parenthood is the only source of free or low-cost women's health screening services in the area." This might have been true years or decades before—now, however, it wasn't.

Particularly disconcerting was the statement that "Komen and its Affiliates do not provide any funding for abortions or for any activities outside the scope of our promise to end breast cancer." Certainly, it was true that no Komen dollars were supposed to go to abortion, but the reality is, we had no way to really know. In fact, as I looked into the grants further, it would turn out that in several Planned Parenthood grants, funds could be used for general administrative overhead or for salaries of certain employees.

I am not suggesting that Komen was intentionally trying to mislead anyone. Rather, I am pointing out *why* Komen was moving in the direction that it was with its granting program. Clearly, higher standards and stricter criteria made good sense for an organization investing such significant dollars in so many programs.

———

Komen had reached a decision point. The organization was entering its thirtieth year. Fund-raising was tougher and more competitive than ever. Expectations were higher—from our donors and our board. The Planned Parenthood issue was not going away. The quality of the grants would have to be addressed at some point—the evolution of the granting strategy was going to happen; it was just a question of timing. Planned Parenthood's controversies were affecting fund-raising, and managing the fallout from their issues was a major distraction for us and a drain on manpower.

It came down to this: Were the Planned Parenthood grants so impactful, so critical to our mission and the woman we serve, that we would continue to take the negative PR hits, expend valuable staff time managing issues that were not ours, and lose significant fund-raising opportunities?

3

The Gathering Storm

Komen began the initiative to change the way community grants were selected and awarded in early 2010. We wanted real results—results that could be measured beyond just the number of women who attended a breast health education program. After all, women attending seminars wasn't really saving lives. We wanted our work to affect the actual health of women—to reduce the number of late-stage diagnoses and increase breast cancer survival rates.

Komen affiliates were now required to conduct an intensive "community assessment" to identify needs in their community, and the grants they awarded were supposed to address these needs. This process was part of evolving our strategy and provided new focus for the affiliates as they determined which grants to award.

It was clear that general education and awareness grants were not high-impact programs. This is not to say that education and awareness are unimportant. Komen awarded millions for these types of grants—re-funding the same or similar programs year after year. Scores of grants—perhaps even hundreds—focused on culturally appropriate education and outreach. But the quality and success of these programs varied greatly from community to community, and it was expensive to fund the creation of language-specific materials repeatedly. It made more sense to create a national library of these types of programs. Komen National would develop these programs, using proven strategies and the latest approaches. The Circle of Promise, geared toward African-American women, had already been launched, and Lazos que Perduran (Bonds That Last), to reach Latina women, would be next.

Additionally, Komen was moving away from "pass-through" type grants—where one organization received the grant but paid another organization to actually provide the service. To the greatest extent possible, Komen would grant to the organization that actually delivered the service.

It is important to note that this shift in strategies, and the more stringent eligibility and performance standards to support them, were not specifically developed because of or directed at Planned Parenthood—or any other organization, for that matter. We believed that this new strategy would increase the quality and consistency, as well as the impact, of our grants. At the same time, we could do it in a much more cost-effective way—freeing up significant dollars that would be invested in other community programs, to serve even more women.

There was a growing awareness that Komen's efforts to strengthen our granting would affect the Planned Parenthood grants. Liz even specifically mentioned the poor quality of the Planned Parenthood education grants on the very first conference call regarding Planned Parenthood in which I participated as a new Komen employee. Under the revised granting strategy, most of the Planned Parenthood grants would not qualify.

But it is also important to acknowledge that Komen was also looking for an exit strategy for the Planned Parenthood grants. Komen had been under fire about Planned Parenthood for years, and the heat was intensifying. As we explored our options to transition out of our relationship with Planned Parenthood, various possibilities were identified and evaluated. I was specifically tasked with identifying these possibilities. Obviously, if indeed the Planned Parenthood grants were "crappy," as Liz had called them, the new grant direction provided a reasonable and rational off-ramp. In the end, however, the decision rested with Liz and Nancy, with the board's agreement.

Gathering Steam

The election of 2010 was clearly a turning point—with sweeping successes for the GOP. The pro-life community engaged seriously in contests across the country. Taking cues from the left, it was becoming more sophisticated and aggressive.

There was also little doubt that the pro-life community wanted to stop President Obama from enacting his far-left social agenda. The Catholic Church assumed a more forceful and public posture in the political arena as well. President Obama and a Democratic Congress were erasing the gains of the past decade. And this was fueling the pro-life groups' commitment. An executive order from President Bush had prevented taxpayers from funding abortions

abroad. President Obama rolled back that executive order immediately upon entering office. President George W. Bush had issued
an executive order preventing federal funding for most lines of
embryonic stem cell research. President Obama immediately did
away with that, too. Meanwhile, pro-life groups and activists were
employing new legislative and legal tactics to battle abortion clinics. New zoning laws affecting abortion clinics were being implemented. A number of states passed laws prohibiting state money
to any organizations that provided abortion on demand. Several
governors used executive orders, budget vetoes, or new contract
rules to bar state funds for Planned Parenthood.

The outcry surrounding Planned Parenthood began to spike
at the beginning of 2011. Congressman Mike Pence (R-IN) introduced a bill to end federal funding for Planned Parenthood altogether. Pence stated, "The largest abortion provider in America
should not also be the largest recipient of federal funding under
Title X."

In February 2011, Lila Rose and her group Live Action released undercover videos from inside Planned Parenthood. The
videos depicted the manager of a New Jersey clinic explaining to
two individuals, one posing as a pimp and the other an underage
prostitute, how to apply for government services. "The only thing
that you do have to be careful is if they are a minor we are obligated if we hear any certain information to kind of report," the
manager told the Live Action journalists. "So as long as they just
lie and say, 'Oh he's fifteen, sixteen.' You know, as long as they
don't say 'fourteen' and as long as it's not too much of an age gap
then we just kind of like play it [stupid]." Rose said, "This proves

beyond a shadow of a doubt that Planned Parenthood intentionally breaks state and federal laws and covers up the abuse of the
young girls it claims to serve."

Cecile Richards, president of Planned Parenthood Federation
of America, said in a letter to U.S. Attorney General Eric Holder
that the Live Action video may have been "a hoax." But even
Planned Parenthood had to admit that the behavior was "inappropriate."[1] Pressure grew for action on Planned Parenthood.

In March, when this story hit *Philanthropy Today*, Komen's
anxiety increased. Was the Planned Parenthood clinic exposed in
the video a Komen grantee? Fortunately, it was not, but the incident put the Planned Parenthood issue back on the front burner,
with Nancy requesting an assessment of the situation.

While I was made aware of Nancy's request, I was not yet a
Komen employee and was not involved in the meetings. Mollie
Williams was tasked with reviewing options together with other
department heads. She prepared a summary of the discussion
and presented the group's recommendation. Details of this meeting and the resulting recommendation were leaked to the press.[2]
The recommendation was to maintain the status quo. I would
later learn that the rationale was that those who oppose Komen's
funding to Planned Parenthood will never rest until all funding
to the organization is stopped and that it was a slippery slope
to base granting decisions on politics. The bias toward Planned
Parenthood—rather than Komen's best interest—was evident
to me. Why was there an assumption that anything was being
based on politics? To me, the essential questions should have
always focused on the quality of grants and the overall impact to

Komen. Politics was never part of my thought process, and I was surprised to see it referenced as part of the thought process in this initial assessment.

Meanwhile, Planned Parenthood remained a hot topic in Congress—and in the media.

On February 18, 2011, the U.S. House of Representatives, by a vote of 240–185, voted to defund Planned Parenthood. The issue went to the U.S. Senate.

By the end of February, mammograms—and consequently Komen—were brought into the Planned Parenthood controversy. Under siege and facing the possibility of losing hundreds of millions of dollars in federal funding—a significant percentage of Planned Parenthood's overall revenue—Cecile went on the offensive. She appeared on Joy Behar's show on HLN to plead her case. If Congress cut off funding to Planned Parenthood, Cecile said, women would lose access "not to abortion services, (but) to basic family planning, you know, mammograms."[3] Investigative journalist Lila Rose began calling Planned Parenthood clinics around the country and discovered that Planned Parenthood does not provide mammograms. The story was picked up widely in the media. Pro-life groups were direct: Cecile was lying.

But Cecile had found a compelling message. It didn't matter that Planned Parenthood didn't provide mammograms. By linking itself to the fight against breast cancer, Planned Parenthood could shift the debate away from abortion—and focus the debate on something that most would support. Planned Parenthood would soon launch an aggressive campaign hitching itself to the issue of breast cancer—using the hot pink that had long been associated with breast cancer whenever possible.

This would pull Komen deeper into a debate that we had no desire to be in.

***

As Planned Parenthood's mammogram controversy continued through March, Nancy would again point out that this was a fight that Komen did not need to be in. She thanked me for continuing to monitor the situation and said that Komen needed to act; that we should either simply ignore or get out of the grants with Planned Parenthood and identify direct providers for mammograms and other breast health services. She also noted that we were spending a tremendous amount of time on an issue that was not ours.

My official first day with Komen was April 4. My first official meeting on Planned Parenthood was April 6.

Liz called the meeting, despite the fact that there had just been a similar meeting the month before. That we were meeting again seemed to me to indicate that concerns had heightened since the last formal discussion on the issue. The participants included Liz, Mollie, Katrina, Leslie, and two Komen board members. One was from Colorado and was the affiliate representative to the board; the other was longtime Democratic lobbyist John Raffaelli. We discussed the grants process and the importance of maintaining the integrity of that process. I learned that Komen grants were awarded based on an independent, competitive process. This was good, but I still had questions—details that I needed to understand in order to effectively meet Nancy's request that options be identified. Did all nineteen grants to Planned Parenthood rank the highest? I challenged the statement that

Planned Parenthood was the only provider in some areas. Did we know this to be fact? Had we ever explored alternative providers? After all, we were talking about only nineteen grants, and most of them were in major urban areas.

The lobbyist board member jumped in. He went through various decision points, including ending the funding altogether or narrowing the number of grants. Then he added, "No matter what we do, it's not enough. These groups would rather see people die than go to Planned Parenthood." I was shocked that a board member would make such a politically charged statement.

It was during this call that I first heard Liz talk about the direction she wanted to take our grants. She made the point that most of the Planned Parenthood grants were education grants and questioned the value of continuing to re-grant these same types of programs over and over. Liz also raised her own broader concerns about Planned Parenthood—noting that the organization seemed not to know its mission, and calling the mammography focus "not honest."

Leslie Aun, Komen's new communications vice president, noted that Planned Parenthood was "under the gun" and that if Komen ended the grants, our organization would deal Planned Parenthood "a body blow." I could not believe what I was hearing. Why was it our problem or our issue what happened to Planned Parenthood? Our concern was for our organization and our mission.

As the call wrapped up, Liz went through next steps. The current Planned Parenthood grants were to be reviewed and, as we moved forward with the new granting model, education grants would be limited. My notes from this call reference that Liz specifically said Komen would consider tabling the grants until Planned Parenthood figured out just what type of organization it was.

But the issue would linger without a definitive decision on our direction for some months.

Some conservatives were calling for boycotts against the American Cancer Society (ACS) Relay for Life, because of the society's links with organizations that provided abortions and conducted embryonic stem cell research.[4] Despite Nancy's concerns—and those of others, including me—many within Komen remained dismissive, seeing no threat at all to our organization. One member of the communications team—John Hammarley, who would later become a press source—noted that the targeting of the American Cancer Society at least meant that Komen wasn't alone in being in the pro-life crosshairs.

The comment made me uncomfortable—not because of the issues. Rather, because I felt as though there was a sense of joy in Komen's having company and that it was somehow a badge of honor to be a target. For me, the real issue was that Komen should not be in anyone's crosshairs. Komen was about one thing: breast cancer.

I made my views on this known, stating very directly that we needed to stay focused on supporting access for women to breast health services; that we should not be for or against either side.

In April, the Indiana Legislature passed a bill barring

Planned Parenthood from state funding. Governor Mitch Dan-
iels signed the bill into law. Other states would follow.

Next, Senator David Vitter (R-LA) weighed in on the issue.
We saw this for what it is. Facing a tough reelection, Vitter was
using the tried-and-true campaign tactic for conservatives—
say you are the most pro-life and everything will be fine. We
thanked the senator and his wife for their longtime support.
While Mollie advocated that we extol the virtues of Planned
Parenthood and the grants, we responded politely, seeing no reason to inflame matters further.

It was now July, and the abortion and stem cell issues were
as hot as the record-breaking temperatures in Dallas that summer. Some religious groups worried about Komen's position—did
Komen support research using human embryos or not? These
worries were heightened by a five-year-old Komen newsletter
that cited the possibilities of breakthroughs via embryonic stem
cell research and was still on the Komen website. Then a media
report included comments from a Komen spokesperson that
were interpreted to mean that Komen was open to this type of
research. I was at a loss. Komen had never funded embryonic
stem cell research and had no plans to do so. I could not understand why our statement didn't just stop there. Speculating about
the future made no sense, especially since this type of research
held virtually no promise for breast cancer and Komen had not
even received applications for this area of research. The comments were based on a previously developed press statement, and
unfortunately, this dated statement was used without a recent
review.[5]

The Catholic Backlash

By July, Komen was in the middle of a firestorm.

Bishop Leonard Blair of Toledo, Ohio, was the first to act. "In order to avoid even the possibility of cooperation in morally unacceptable activities," he wrote in his statement, "the other Bishops and I believe that it would be wise to find alternatives to Komen for Catholic fundraising efforts."[6]

We responded to Bishop Blair, trying to persuade him. I was asked to work with the communications team to craft the response for our Ohio affiliate. The response pointed out that local Catholic hospitals had received more than $1.3 million from Komen affiliates and that Komen had never funded abortion or embryonic stem cell research. We further noted that in the last year, Catholic hospitals and other faith-based organizations had received more than two hundred Komen grants.[7]

A few weeks later, the bishops of the Catholic Conference of Ohio issued a statement to "direct Catholic parishes and schools away from fundraising for Komen for the Cure and toward activities and organizations that are fully consistent with Catholic moral teaching." The conference specifically cited our "financial contributions to Planned Parenthood. . . . The Ohio Bishops reaffirmed the Church's commitment to human life and health, and to the dignity of the human person at all stages of development. They expressed a common desire to avoid even indirect support for research involving human embryos."[8]

The Catholic Conference of Ohio stopped just short of a full condemnation. At least, individual Catholics could continue to support Komen. Still, it was a public relations disaster and it was spreading across the country, one diocese to the next, and generating significant media coverage.

The press coverage was extensive and less than optimal. It was one thing to be targeted about Planned Parenthood, but Komen did not and had not funded embryonic stem cell research. It seemed a stretch for the Ohio bishops to target Komen about something that it might perhaps do in the future. Komen gave substantial funds to faith-based organizations—far more than Planned Parenthood received—and the overwhelming majority of those were Catholic. In just a single year, Komen had awarded nearly three hundred grants, totaling close to $17 million.

Liz and Katrina dissected the bishops' letter and seemed to think that the church's motives were more about fund-raising. As for me, I didn't think it mattered what the reason was behind the bishops' decision. This was the Catholic Church, and a full-scale national boycott would have severe consequences for Komen.

The fallout continued. Team captains for races around the nation were weighing in—by unregistering. In a two-day period, one Komen affiliate lost two Catholic schools that had participated in numerous previous races. This was on top of losing sponsorships from several local banks and losing a major grocery store sponsor to another event. The affiliate noted that this would take a dent out of its fund-raising.

More bishops joined with Ohio. And some went further,

advising even individual parishioners not to support Komen. Komen was even a topic at Mass on several Sundays.

In Ohio, the lieutenant governor backed out of the race.

At the end of July, Gallup released a new poll on abortion and government funding for Planned Parenthood. It underscored the deep division in our country on the issues.

Our affiliates were anxious and overwhelmed. National had to do something, they begged. A new session specifically to discuss these issues was hastily added to the annual Presidents and Executive Directors Forum. The leadership from scores of affiliates attended. The room was overflowing—with people and emotion. I remember several references to "Crazy Catholics" and "nutty right-wingers." One Komen affiliate representative was reduced to tears. Some in the room said that Komen's mission trumped all others, and if the Planned Parenthood grants were hurting the organization, it was time to walk away. This infuriated others who said that a woman's right to choose had to be protected at any and all costs—even if Komen suffered.

The tenor of this meeting and the deep split within our own ranks reinforced my belief that Komen was, as Nancy had said repeatedly, in the middle of a fight that was not ours. We had to find a way to get to neutral ground. I recommended to Liz that it was time to consider go-forward strategies. Liz agreed.

However, we would not discuss the issue formally again until early September. By this time, we had agreed that reevaluating our embryonic stem cell statement made sense. This type of research had shown little to no promise for breast cancer. Why fight a fight for something that was not relevant to our mission?

With this clarified position, we would take one volatile issue off the table for ourselves.

In our discussion about Planned Parenthood, I presented various possible alternatives. The first was to "continue as is." I made the point—as I would do repeatedly in the coming months—that this was an option. I also proposed that we consider revising Komen's policy, so that a donor could direct that no part of the contribution would go to Planned Parenthood. I noted that large organizations like the United Way were doing so. This went nowhere. One option was also a general exclusionary policy— simply say we would not grant to Planned Parenthood because of the controversies. This was discussed and quickly rejected. We also discussed how the revised grants process and updated criteria might affect Planned Parenthood and whether this would be an appropriate resolution.

This meeting concluded with no definitive decision on what direction to take.

As the issue developed, the Komen Board of Directors was also kept up to date on the challenges the organization was facing, and those challenges were growing.

Across the country, thirty-six Komen affiliates in twenty-seven states were working to address concerns regarding Planned Parenthood and embryonic stem-cell research. Significant resources and goodwill were being diverted from our breast cancer work to managing these issues. The political landscape would keep the Planned Parenthood issue front and center. It seemed to me—and Nancy and Liz said they agreed—that we were expending a significant amount of time and energy on the issue that could—and should—be spent on fighting breast cancer.

Our chief goal, I pointed out, had to be deescalating the situation with the Catholic Church and preventing "spillover" with other religious organizations.

I was asked to develop and present potential "next steps" that could be effective in calming the controversy. Obviously, we were continuing to move toward the implementation of outcomes-based granting, and as this was rolled out, various types of grants, including those with Planned Parenthood, would be affected. With a more definitive statement on the embryonic stem cell issue, we had an opportunity to reach out to the faith-based community.

None of the recommendations involved cutting off funding for Planned Parenthood.

Promise Me

As if fending off the Catholic community and other pro-lifers weren't enough, that summer Komen's Promise Me perfume would create a stink—quite literally. The launch of the perfume was a big deal for Nancy. She was even on a segment on the Home Shopping Network.

But the perfume brought out Komen critics. Breast Cancer Action, a longtime Komen rival and detractor with a long history of questioning Komen's marketing practices, said this was another example of Komen being a corporate sellout and that "pinkwashing," as it was called, was hurting the fight against breast cancer. While the Operating Committee was not briefed on the perfume issues, I was not immediately concerned. But when the *USA Today* picked up on the story and I read the accusation that the perfume contained ingredients that were said to be linked to breast cancer in lab animals, I was alarmed.[9] Soon letters were pouring into Komen's offices decrying Promise Me, taking Komen to task, saying that women should not have to worry whether our products were bad for their health—especially those with pink ribbons on them.

Next, *Pink Ribbons, Inc.,* an explosive documentary making the case that the pink ribbon campaign had actually hurt the fight against breast cancer, made its debut in September at the Toronto International Film Festival.[10] Nancy and Komen were featured prominently.

The Problems Escalate

I didn't think things could get any worse. But they did.

October, which is National Breast Cancer Awareness Month, was obviously an important time for Komen. But we were engulfed in controversy.

Affiliates were still struggling with the significant backlash from the Planned Parenthood grants. Many reported that it was having a significant effect on donations. One affiliate executive director actually pleaded with Komen to stop funding Planned Parenthood, because she felt that we were losing race participants and donations because of it.

The panic seemed palpable from affiliates across the country.

We did have our supporters, of course. The bishop of Alexandria, Louisiana, wrote that his parishioners could be confident that Komen wasn't funding Planned Parenthood's abortions, and that the Catholic faith-based health-care facility Christus St. Frances Cabrini Hospital was proud to be a major sponsor of the local race.

But this was the exception, not the rule. Iowa Right to Life suggested that Komen was closely tied to Planned Parenthood. This prompted the Komen affiliate there to ask about a proactive plan to address the issues. In Jacksonville, Florida, on the eve of the big Georgia-Florida college football game, a billboard on a major highway read: "Susan G. Komen for the Cure Supports Planned Parenthood."

The Tipping Point

Senator Marco Rubio (R-FL), a rising Tea Party star, was a strong advocate for Komen. He and his family participated in the October 15 Race for the Cure in Miami, and Senator and Mrs. Rubio had agreed to serve as honorary chairmen of Komen's Perfect Pink Party in Palm Beach, Nancy's home. The senator announced his race participation on Twitter the morning of the race. The tweet created a Twitter backlash that prompted his chief of staff to contact a Komen board member and then me.

My concern at this point was less about the grants themselves and more about Komen's credibility and our obligation for full disclosure about them. Nancy had recently met with the senator but the issue was not addressed. I knew from following Senator Rubio's career that he is extremely pro-life, and I was certain that this had to be a difficult issue for him—his desire to support Komen versus his faith. I would later learn that the senator received calls from two Florida bishops.

A week later, the senator withdrew from Komen, including stepping away from his role with the Palm Beach gala in January. I was not surprised. Nor did I relish having to tell Nancy.

Nancy did not seem to take it well at all, and I don't blame her. We just lost the participation of an influential senator, and the issue would now likely bring even more questions from the Hill. I don't think Nancy was angry at Senator Rubio; she understood his situation. I think she was angry that Komen continued to be caught in the middle of an issue that was not ours.

That same day, we got word that our corporate partners were being hit about Komen's relationship with Planned Parenthood. Chain letters were making their way to corporate donors, including our biggest partners. The letters claimed that we were deeply involved with Planned Parenthood and that the abortions funded by Planned Parenthood raised the risk of breast cancer. At the same time, emails that the Komen Help Desk had sent that directed women to Planned Parenthood were circulating on the Internet.

It seemed that frustrations were high. Liz told me she wanted to come out swinging. Nancy seemed to just want to be done with it all. I did my best to calm everyone and reiterate that it really was time to make a decision one way or the other.

The Planned Parenthood issue was nearly consuming the organization. I was spending more than half of my time dealing with it—working with the communications team and the affiliates to address the questions and concerns.

While the pro-life backlash and the Promise Me issue were bad, it was the situation with Senator Rubio that weighed most heavily.

In 2010, Komen had received about one thousand emails on Planned Parenthood. So far in 2011, the volume of negative emails had increased nearly 50 percent—and this was just through the end of October.

Our affiliates continued to do their best to deal with the issue. In early November, an affiliate advised that a major sponsor pulled out. The loss represented significant dollars and hundreds of race participants. Trying to determine if this was an isolated incidence, she said that it didn't take much digging to identify tens of thousands of dollars in lost donations. She said that race donations and walkers were down substantially. The local TV sponsor even had to take down its Facebook posting because of the backlash.

Nancy left for a two-week trip out of the country at the end of October. While she was away, I was directed to review the previously discussed options regarding Planned Parenthood, fine-tune them if needed, and redistribute. Nancy, it seemed, was ready to move forward. The only issue that remained was exactly how we would do that.

In early November, we started to see the Planned Parenthood effect on Komen's 3-Day race. The event director expressed concerns, and this seemed to get Katrina's attention.

December brought still more controversy. The Bible printer LifeWay Christian Resources, a division of the Southern Baptist Convention's publishing house, came under fire for its partnership with Komen. The partnership involved the Here's Hope Breast Cancer Bible—with a bright pink cover. The Bible was being sold at Wal-Mart and other retailers, with a dollar from each sale coming back to Komen. The backlash was immediate. Susan Tyrrell of LifeNews.com wrote, "The sign might as well read, 'Buy a Bible and support abortion!' "[11]

A marketing initiative with the Bible? I really had a hard time understanding this. More importantly, though, I wondered why, with all that we were facing, this initiative had not been brought up. This would not only reignite the faith-based organizations, but it would fuel our detractors who already felt that Komen cheapened the fight against breast cancer by "pinking" so many products.

LifeWay quickly responded, "We made a mistake." "Though we have assurances that Komen's funds are used only for breast cancer screening and awareness," said Thom Rainer, president of LifeWay, "it is not in keeping with LifeWay's core values to have even an indirect relationship with Planned Parenthood."[12] The pink Bibles would be recalled.

And so it was decided—it was time to implement our plan.

If we thought that the pro-life side was tough, we had no idea what was in store from President Obama, Planned Parenthood, and the organized left. And I had no idea that the coincidences would become so prevalent, I would begin to wonder if Planned Parenthood had some inside help.

4

Planned Infiltration

Why did it take until the end of 2011 to make a decision Komen had been pursuing since before I joined? I'm not sure, but I think it was because Nancy and Liz—and even Komen generally— were deeply conflicted about Planned Parenthood and the grants.

To understand why, you have to understand Nancy—and Komen—a bit better.

━━━━━

Nancy is formidable. She has a true iron will—and usually gets what she wants one way or another. Nancy also has detractors, and they were usually eager to share, although almost always hidden behind the curtain of "a person familiar with the situation." But most hard-charging, assertive women have critics—I knew this firsthand. I admired Nancy for all that she had accomplished in her career and in the fight against breast cancer—and I still do. That is not to say that I didn't understand why some might find her and Komen difficult.

She preferred to be addressed as Ambassador Brinker. I'd read the claims of her wanting to be known as the "Duchess of Boobs." That seems ridiculous—I never heard her use that phrase. She is a serious woman on a serious mission, and I can't imagine her demeaning herself or Komen in that way.

Some saw Nancy as self-serving. I saw her more as politically astute. She knows that portraying herself as apolitical keeps her part of the "in" crowd—regardless of which crowd is in. She is a political pragmatist, able to straddle the political fence with ease—and for a purpose: to advance Komen's mission.

She moves as easily among Democrats as Republicans. And she has the credibility to do so.

She sat on the board of Planned Parenthood of North Texas in 2002. In 2010 she wrote and released her memoir. President Obama was in the White House and Democrats controlled Congress. In what I thought was probably not a coincidence, she recounted a situation from 2004 in which the women's fitness company Curves withdrew its support because of Komen's affiliation with Planned Parenthood. "The grants in question supplied breast health counseling, screening, and treatments to rural women, poor women, Native American women, many women of color who were underserved—if served at all—in areas where Planned Parenthood facilities were often the only infrastructure available," Nancy wrote. "Though it meant losing corporate money from Curves, we were not about to turn our back on these women. Somehow this position translated to the utterly false assertion that SGK funds abortions."[1]

That was Nancy—shoring up her political credibility with the new "in" crowd.

It worked.

Soon after the book was released, President Obama presented Nancy with the Presidential Medal of Freedom.

As I said, I admire Nancy. She does what she must in her pursuit of a world without breast cancer—and to keep her promise to her sister Suzy. When Nancy founded Komen, the five-year survival rate for breast cancer was just 74 percent. Today it's nearly 98 percent. "I was raised in the era of polio," Nancy told *Hadassah* magazine. "The country marshaled all its resources and all but eradicated polio. Maybe breast cancer will have the same chance."[2] In the fight against cancer, there can be no doubt that Nancy Goodman Brinker has changed lives and saved lives.

Some viewed Nancy as a bit self-absorbed, leaving those around her sometimes feeling hurt and unappreciated. But I suppose in a number of ways, this was an example of how singularly focused she was.

Nancy is tough—something I didn't mind. She also can be thin-skinned sometimes, it seemed to me especially when it came to press coverage.

Komen was an organization in transition, evolving from a start-up nonprofit to a thirty-year-old global force and working to strengthen its infrastructure and leadership. Turnover was a challenge, and because of the turnover, there sometimes was a lack of continuity and consistency—in processes and practices and how they were applied.[3]

However, Komen is one of the most respected organizations in the country—a fund-raising juggernaut that had earned the coveted four-star ranking from Charity Navigator multiple years in a row.

Komen's structure could be unwieldy for an organization of its size, and I felt there was ambiguity between Nancy's role as CEO and Liz Thompson's as president, making it difficult to know who actually made the decisions.

As Komen entered its thirtieth year, Nancy knew that the organization had to change. That's why the initiative to move to a more outcomes-based granting model was launched. But it was more than that. Komen's structure, with nearly 130 separate affiliates, was outdated and expensive. A major organization-wide initiative to restructure Komen by consolidating the local affiliates and National into a single, consolidated entity, with fewer affiliates and local races was launched. Long-term, this would create a stronger, more efficient and more cohesive Komen. Short-term, these strategic shifts would fuel the animosity and distrust that many affiliates had against the national operation— another factor that would play into future events.

At the same time, the financial picture was increasingly cloudy. The poor economic climate made for an uncertain consumer. The affiliates were struggling with their races—much of which they attributed to Planned Parenthood. Some corporate partnerships had also been lost and other areas of fund-raising were hurting—some, no doubt, as a result of Planned Parenthood as well. After the 2010 and 2011 Global Race for the Cure, held in June in Washington, D.C., experienced a downward trend in participants, a major retooling was begun.

We had a lot on our plate and the controversies surrounding Planned Parenthood were adding to it.

Decision Time

Nancy now wanted to move, and fast. It wasn't just Rubio's withdrawal, the pink Bible fiasco, and the internal demands of managing the Planned Parenthood liabilities. It was the combined weight of all the issues—the perfume, new questions about Komen's marketing practices, the critical *Pink Ribbons, Inc.* film, fund-raising challenges, and friction between National and the affiliates. How much could the organization withstand? Komen was trying to keep a lot of balls in the air—financial concerns, organizational changes, global expansion—while also managing the fallout from various other public relations issues. Something had to give—and that something was Planned Parenthood.

On August 17, 2011, one of Nancy's confidants at Komen relayed her desire to move more quickly. Apparently Nancy was growing more and more frustated. When word began circulating that Nancy had been a board member for Planned Parenthood of North Texas and received an award from them in 1997, Nancy seemed exasperated, saying that Planned Parenthood had been using her name long after she had asked that it be removed.

Planned Parenthood continued to consume our time, and Nancy became more and more adamant that it was time to make a decision.

Meanwhile, Liz seemed to vacillate. One minute, she appeared to be annoyed that Planned Parenthood was even an issue. The next minute, she seemed frustrated and angry, especially since the Planned Parenthood grants were "crappy" in the first place. Liz even said, at one point, that she thought we had to try to get out of the culture wars.

And this back-and-forth would continue. Meetings were held. Liz and Nancy discussed. But still there was no decision one way or the other.

Liz and I never discussed our personal views on abortion and life—in fact, there was never any discussion of anyone's personal beliefs on these issues. Still, I sensed that Liz was genuinely conflicted, not because the Planned Parenthood grants were impactful to our mission—she'd repeatedly said they were not. Rather, she seemed to be trying to reconcile her beliefs with what was best for Komen. Liz's friendship with Cecile may have also contributed to her angst. Liz would say that she and Cecile Richards, head of Planned Parenthood, had known each other for years, regularly sitting on panels together. I had the impression that Liz held Cecile in high regard.

The other players at Komen seemed generally against any action that would affect Planned Parenthood, but not because of the women we served or the quality of the grants.

Katrina McGhee was an ardent and vocal opponent. But she didn't seem to care about the grants and whether they were impactful. She seemed most concerned about whether ending the grants would create an "uprising from the left" that would further affect revenues. However, by late fall even Katrina began to recognize the toll the backlash was having, and she began to soften.

Mollie Williams was against transitioning out of the Planned Parenthood grants. To me, her opposition seemed more focused on what this meant for Planned Parenthood than the merit of the grants in the fight against breast cancer. She repeatedly referenced the "sanctity of the grants process," but as I would soon find out, that process was flawed and granting criteria ignored.

Leslie Aun, the communications vice president, was also against the move—she had made that very clear in April when she said any move against Planned Parenthood would deal them "a body blow."

This left me as the person to take the overall lead in coordinating with the relevant function areas across the organization—and carrying out decisions and directions from Nancy and Liz. This was not a political choice. It wasn't even a project I desired. It was simply a matter of personnel. Someone had to take on the task, and I was that person.

I should have realized that I wasn't the right person. I should have known that I was exactly the *wrong* person. I think that Nancy and Liz turned to me for a few reasons. First, it was both a policy and communications issue. Second, I'd been through a firefight with the pro-life groups during my gubernatorial campaign. And third, I had already proven that I could get even difficult tasks done.

However, we failed to consider two key things. First, the politics of it all. Liz and Nancy knew, as I did, that no one's personal ideology drove the decision. The decision was made in the best interest of Komen and the women we served. We knew we could achieve better results by redirecting the Planned Parenthood dollars to other higher-impact programs. In awarding grants to Planned Parenthood, we were caught in the middle of a divisive ideological and political debate. As a result, we were facing a strong, sustained backlash and were cut off from a significant source of potential revenue. We were trying to extricate ourselves and put Komen in a position to be supported by everyone— regardless of their views on abortion.

As we worked through the decision, our mission and the women we served were always the top priority. If anyone really believed that ending the grants would have left women without critical breast health services, I am convinced that we would have stayed the course. But this was not raised as a concern because there were alternatives. These grants were inconsequential to Komen's mission and they were inconsequential to Planned Parenthood's mission.

I knew that some would view our decision through a political lens—and I'm sure that others realized this, too—but we knew our motives were pure. Rightly, wrongly, naïvely—we genuinely believed that others would see the reasonableness of our actions and understand, as Nancy had said many times, "we had no dog in this fight."

The second thing we failed to consider? That I would actually get the job done.

We had no dog in this fight, and we were determined that neither side of the debate would be able to claim a scalp. This was our guiding principle.

In early November, Katrina informed Nancy that the Planned Parenthood challenges were now affecting the 3-Day race. I followed up that the issue had been hurting Komen at the community level for months. We had tried to manage the issue with messaging about how little Komen gave to Planned Parenthood, but it was not working. Nancy told me we needed to act, but there was still no decision on *how* we would act. I was asked, once again, to lay out the options for discussion—and, I hoped, a decision.

It seemed that Nancy had made up her mind. She let me know that Komen would need to fundamentally disengage from poor grants, including those with Planned Parenthood. She wanted a policy that all grants, at both the community and national level, would meet the highest standards. She pointed out that it was not Komen's job to manage Planned Parenthood's public relations. She also acknowledged that the controversy was affecting fund-raising and taking us away from our mission. She did not want to yield to anger but she saw the damage it was doing to Komen. She reinforced that our mission was the priority.

I responded that we were in total agreement that our mission must come first. I also specifically noted, once again, that if the Planned Parenthood grants met Komen's goal of delivering exceptional grants, I understood.

"Moving to Neutral Ground"

On November 7, I presented four options to Nancy and Liz. They were: 1) transition to the outcomes-based granting model and, as a result, transition out of the Planned Parenthood grants; 2) exclude certain organizations from being eligible for Komen grants; 3) simply end the Planned Parenthood grants as of December

31—a hard stop, if you will; and 4) stay the course and continue granting to Planned Parenthood as Komen had been doing for years.

———

The goal was to move to "neutral ground"—to keep politics away from Komen and Komen out of politics. I provided the pros and cons of each option in full detail. After my meeting with Liz and Nancy, my understanding was that they wanted to move forward with a "hard stop," ending all Planned Parenthood grants as of December 31. I agreed with that approach.

The Dance of Indecision

On November 8, the Komen leadership met to discuss our options. Liz joined by phone. Nancy didn't attend—she was still traveling. The rest of us gathered in the fifth-floor conference room in Dallas.

I began walking through the options. When I reached the third option—ending the grants to Planned Parenthood—Katrina pushed back. I asked Liz if she wanted to add her thoughts.

When Liz spoke, I did not expect her words. She waffled, going into the integrity of the grants process once again. I pushed back, thinking that perhaps Liz was trying to invite more debate to ensure that everyone's thoughts were on the table.

I continued to hold my ground, making the case I thought I had been directed to make. Finally, Katrina said, "Karen, what don't you understand about what the president is telling you?"

The room went silent. The tone was angry and demeaning. Her implication clear to everyone—that I was insubordinate, foolish, and completely misguided regarding Planned Parenthood.

I was proceeding as both Liz and Nancy had asked. If Nancy and Liz wanted to stay the course, so be it. At least we would finally know where we were going, which would mean we could all plan accordingly—for fund-raising, communications, policy, and with our affiliates. I was frustrated that there was still no decision. Continuing to dwell in the mushy space of indecisiveness was untenable and even more damaging for Komen.

I decided to just let it go. I would go back to Nancy and Liz for additional guidance—perhaps they'd changed their minds. Nancy emailed me the following day to reassure me that a decision would be made.

I let Nancy know that I was deeply troubled by the entire exchange. I proceeded as I thought they wanted me to—only to be thrown under the bus.

A few days later, on November 9, I got word from Nancy, who was still out of the country, that she had had time and distance to think through the issues and that she wanted to be done for good with Planned Parenthood.

I hoped that we finally had a decision, but that would not be the case.

The office seemed to be fracturing, with those who were against the move pushing back directly to Nancy and Liz. We were now back to square one. Nancy asked about getting real research that showed American opinion. I thought this probably came through Katrina, who looked to marketing surveys for most things. Nancy also said she wanted a thorough, objective study of present grant outcomes and alternative providers. I thought this probably was Mollie's suggestion. Nancy and I were both concerned that the organization seemed to be dividing into camps.

The endless discussion and temporizing were frustrating. I thought Nancy's goal was for Komen to be on "neutral ground" by January 1. We could certainly complete market research on public opinion quickly, but there was already a significant amount of research on the subject—all of which pointed to the deep division and volatility that exists around Planned Parenthood and abortion. It was unrealistic that a detailed study of outcomes from the current grants could be completed in time to meet that timeline. It was my understanding that Komen had already done some of this analysis—how else would Nancy and Liz have come to the conclusion that Komen needed to focus more on outcomes? Besides, Liz had been saying for months that education and pass-through grants did not meet the higher standards that we would demand. The call for more studies seemed to me to be stall tactics.

I wasn't going to let Nancy—or anyone else for that matter—get the impression that I was ramming through a position that she herself had endorsed and then find myself being blamed because of my personal politics. My frustrations finally boiled over in an email to Nancy in which I said that I realized some were trying to make this about politics—more specifically, my politics and even my religion. I told Nancy that anyone making these allegations would be wrong and that the motives and biases of those making such comments should be considered. I knew that I had looked at the issue objectively and from all sides—as did those who worked with me on the project. We analyzed the risks and presented the options. We obtained input from those who agreed and those who disagreed. We were diligent in always keeping Komen's mission as the top priority.

I also reiterated to Nancy yet again that, in the final analysis, the question was this: are the Planned Parenthood grants so important, so impactful to the mission that we should make this the hill to climb and potentially die on? If the answer is yes, that's fine. We just needed to make a decision one way or the other and develop our plan forward accordingly.

Once again, I specifically reminded Nancy that one of her options was to stay the course—to continue as we had with Planned Parenthood.

━━━

Nancy, Liz, and I met on November 15. They informed me that Komen would move forward, but not with an immediate halt to Planned Parenthood's grant as of December 31. Rather, we would begin implementation of the new granting strategy and stricter criteria to support this model, effective January 1, 2012, which would cause a gradual reduction of the Planned Parenthood grants. What I did not know at this time—and I don't think Nancy or Liz realized, either—was that Planned Parenthood was already out of compliance with Komen's existing policies and precedents.

Unplanned Discovery

It was at this point that I began to review Komen's existing granting criteria, standards, and related contracts. I discovered that, under these existing criteria and past precedents, the Planned Parenthood grants should *already* have been halted or, at the very least, have prompted a legal and compliance review. I don't know why no one picked up on the issues. Perhaps it was as simple as no one realizing that Planned Parenthood was out of compliance, rather than Planned Parenthood being given a pass on its contractual obligations. It could also have been symptomatic of Komen's turnover issues, since such turnover can foster inconsistency in any organization. Or, perhaps, it was the organizational structure that gave the local affiliates the authority to manage the grant contracts even though some seemed to lack the expertise to do so effectively. I supposed that it could also have been a well-intentioned desire to avoid rocking the boat on a sensitive issue or even reflective of the loyalties that some Komen affiliates seemed to have for Planned Parenthood. Whatever the reason, Komen's existing contracts and past precedents should have already prompted action on the Planned Parenthood grants.

I compared the requirements that any organization had to meet in order to apply for grants—the eligibility criteria—with the obligations outlined in the actual grant contract. I noticed several inconsistencies.

First, Komen required that its grants could only go to other nonprofit organizations, educational institutions, and government entities. The nonprofit status was a requirement. But the contract that an organization signed upon being awarded the grant allowed for its nonprofit status to be discretionary—that an affiliate "may" terminate a grant if the organization lost its tax-exempt status with the Internal Revenue Service.

The second inconsistency related to an organization's eligibility to receive state or federal government funding. The contract stated clearly that if an organization was debarred from receiving state or federal funds, the organization's grant would be revoked. It was a definitive statement with no discretion and no leeway for mitigating circumstances.

The third seemed to be an even bigger gap. The contractual obligation regarding eligibility to receive government funding was *not* part of the criteria that an organization applying for a grant had to meet. Essentially, this meant that an organization could apply for a grant, and upon receiving the grant, immediately be in violation of the contract.

I am a stickler for details and consistency, so I was immediately concerned. This made no sense to me, and I could not understand how something this important had been overlooked.

These issues were particularly relevant for Planned Parenthood. While Planned Parenthood remained eligible to receive federal funding, the organization had been barred from receiving state government money in several states. For example, New

Jersey governor Christie had signed an executive order barring Planned Parenthood from state funding, and numerous states had enacted legislation that did likewise. Some of the state legislation was in litigation, but at the time, these cases were a moving target, with some of the legislation in force and others under court injunctions preventing implementation. Planned Parenthood and its supporters said that these funding restrictions were political in nature. That was perhaps true—I didn't know the motivation behind each piece of legislation or gubernatorial act. What I did know was that Komen's contract requirements did not address the rationale or motivation behind an organization being barred from government funding.

The grant contract also already included language to address financial and administrative improprieties. The contract said that an organization would be in default if Komen had reasonable good faith to believe that there had been financial or administrative improprieties or fraud by the grantee. This seemed to be a pretty straightforward requirement and there were no qualifiers or definitions related to the types of improprieties. The only issue open to discretion was how "reasonable good faith" was interpreted.

I discussed the situation with legal, and there was consensus that indeed these were inconsistencies. Next, I met with Liz and brought her up to speed on what I had found. It was in this meeting that Liz mentioned, for the first time, Komen's precedent for halting grants under the "reasonable good faith" clause. She specifically cited a situation in which Komen revoked a grant to the Mississippi State Department of Health because of a wide-ranging investigation into "graft," as Liz called it. The Mississippi department remained ineligible for a grant until Komen was satisfied that the issues had been resolved.

This precedent—of having halted grants when an organization was under investigation—is what led to a more detailed discussion regarding various investigations into Planned Parenthood.

The congressional investigation into Planned Parenthood had been launched earlier in the fall, but we had only recently learned about it. I think everyone recognized the political overtone. Still, everyone seemed to share my concerns, especially given the prospects of formal hearings that would no doubt put the Planned Parenthood/mammography issue back in the spotlight.

I was asked to do a little more research regarding Planned Parenthood and any other investigations it might be facing. What I found was disturbing. The volume and scope of investigations into Planned Parenthood were nothing short of shocking. There were dozens of current investigations, pending court actions, formal indictments, and even actual violations of law.

Over the past decade, various state audits of Planned Parenthood had concluded that Planned Parenthood had overbilled for and misused government funds. These states included California, New Jersey, New York, and Washington.[4] And recently, the state of Illinois launched an investigation into Medicaid fraud by a Planned Parenthood chapter in that state. In early 2011, Planned Parenthood itself revoked the affiliations of several clinics in California—because of financial improprieties.[5] Additionally, the Texas attorney general was investigating Planned

Parenthood for Medicare and Medicaid fraud.[6] A grand jury in Johnson County, Kansas, delivered more than one hundred felony and misdemeanor indictments against Planned Parenthood. While the felony counts were dismissed—because key documents went missing under the outgoing administration of Democratic governor Kathleen Sebelius, a matter now also under investigation—the trial regarding dozens of misdemeanor indictments is pending.[7] Further, Planned Parenthood had been found in violation of numerous state laws covering a variety of issues.

No one at Komen was making a judgment regarding Planned Parenthood and the merits of any of the open investigations. But it was a fact that Planned Parenthood had been barred from government funding in some states. It was also a fact that a number of Planned Parenthood chapters had been found in violation of various state laws. It was also a fact that Komen already had a precedent of halting a grant to an organization under investigation—and under far less egregious circumstances. Certainly, some of what Planned Parenthood faced could be viewed as politically motivated. However, that did not diminish the fact that Komen was affiliated with an organization that had deep and serious troubles. We prided ourselves on excellence. Was Planned Parenthood really a grantee of excellence? Would we have continued a partnership with any other organization facing such wide-ranging issues? I thought we would not—as evidenced by the revocation of the Mississippi State Department of Health grant.

Liz directed me to follow up with our legal and audit department. She wanted to know exactly how Komen proceeded in the
case involving Mississippi. After reviewing these circumstances,
it was decided that the revised criteria would address the ambiguity of "reasonable good faith" and spell out clearly and as precisely
as possible what that meant. Liz, Nancy, legal—and I—were all
on the same page about this. *This* is how investigations came to
be added to the criteria—it was not some "right-wing" plot to get
Planned Parenthood. It was appropriate legal and compliance due
diligence on the part of Komen.

Legal developed the specific language. As we worked through
this process, there was significant discussion about the definition
of "investigations." Legal eventually landed on language that
worked. Another significant question involved portability. In
other words, if one hospital in a national network of health-care
facilities was affected, was the entire system affected? This question was posed specifically to Liz, and she said that it should. In
this process, other additional requirements regarding eligibility
and grant revocation were added, underscoring Komen's desire to
have the kind of stringent requirements that granting excellence
required.

━━━━

Nancy and Liz asked that I take the various scenarios for moving forward and run them by Ari Fleischer, who by that time
had been hired by Komen as a kind of communications sounding
board for Nancy and specifically to conduct the search for a new
communications lead.

I told Nancy and Liz that halting the grants because of investigations would be a stopgap and not resolve the larger issue. I also specifically advised that immediately cutting off Planned Parenthood would be a mistake that would very likely ignite a firestorm. I had become convinced that Nancy and Liz had been right from the beginning that the solution was to move forward with the outcomes-based granting approach. I expressed concern about getting into too many details in the press. We should follow the strategy of those organizations that had been successful in transitioning out of Planned Parenthood—focus on our new strategic direction and more stringent requirements. We were changing our granting criteria—organizations do this all the time. Although we wanted an exit strategy from Planned Parenthood, the new criteria were going to be implemented at some point, one way or the other, so it was my view that we avoid making any of this about a specific organization.

However, Liz reinforced the focus on investigations as a rationale for a more immediate end to the relationship with Planned Parenthood. She said that she felt the legal investigation issues would enable Komen to address the Planned Parenthood issue while Komen moved forward with the broader project to streamline the grants process. It seemed to me that Liz was concerned about the breadth of investigations involving Planned Parenthood and the precedent that Komen had already set in revoking a grant for what seemed like far less serious issues.

On November 17, I sent Liz and Nancy an email detailing how Planned Parenthood was out of compliance with our granting criteria. The response I received back said that both Liz and Nancy believed that it was the right approach to ensure compliance and that the next step would be to get communications in order.

However, it is important to underscore that Komen had every contractual basis to simply revoke the Planned Parenthood grants immediately. Yet, despite the fact that Planned Parenthood was already in violation of existing contracts—despite the fact that Komen already had precedent for revoking grants under similar, yet less serious, circumstances—Komen did not do so. Instead, Komen revised the existing contracts to allow Planned Parenthood to regain compliance and ensure that all existing grants could be paid in full.

Effective January 1, Komen would move in a new direction with its community grants and implement more stringent criteria and higher performance standards to support this new model. Planned Parenthood would be ineligible for the time being under these new policies, but it would not be permanently ineligible. Also, while I didn't know at the time what other organizations would be affected, I believed that there would be others, and I believed that everyone else at Komen expected other organizations to be affected as well.

Kid Gloves

When the news of Komen's decision broke, it was portrayed as though Komen was "cutting off" Planned Parenthood—that Komen was making them go cold turkey and, in the process, leaving women stranded without breast health services. Cecile Richards, Planned Parenthood's CEO, even said she was "surprised." None of this was true; yet that's how it was reported. Komen was *never* "cutting off" the Planned Parenthood grants. That was nothing more than Planned Parenthood propaganda, and the media played along. Komen ensured that funding for *all* existing grants through the grant contract period would be provided, and Komen would even continue certain other Planned Parenthood grants, despite the new guidelines. Planned Parenthood knew all of this.

Komen made every effort to work with this longtime partner. I was certain that we were taking steps well beyond those that we would have taken with any other grantee. Based on how Komen proceeded with the state of Mississippi, we were clearly giving more latitude to Planned Parenthood. Komen revised contracts to ensure that Planned Parenthood was back in compliance. For example, the contract with Planned Parenthood of New Jersey was quickly revised so that a January payment could be made on time. At least four Planned Parenthood grants were given exceptions and would continue into the next granting cycle, despite the new criteria. Any grant that already had been awarded for the coming year would also be fulfilled, even though the new strategy and standards were in effect as of January 1, 2012.

Planned Parenthood was treated with the softest of kid gloves. And yet, they seemed to have a sense of entitlement—that their grants existed in perpetuity. No organization was ever guaranteed a renewal of its grants. But just as Planned Parenthood acts as though it is entitled to a never-ending flow of government funding, they seemed to think that their Komen grants were life-time awards.

Komen is a private charitable organization. Komen does not take government funding (with the exception of a handful of license plate revenue sharing programs). This is in stark contrast to Planned Parenthood—which counts on government and our tax dollars for nearly 50 percent of its revenue. Komen had every right—in fact, I would argue, it had a responsibility—to make decisions that were in the organization's best interest, for our mission and the women we served. Komen had the right to pursue programs that it believed yielded the best results and were executed the most efficiently. Komen had every right to move in a new direction—even if that new direction affected a longtime grantee and politically connected organization.

Komen also could have chosen to impose these new standards immediately and across the board with no exceptions whatsoever. We did not—we *chose* not to—for several reasons. Most importantly, we wanted to ensure that there would be no gaps for the women we serve. Further, Komen proceeded with respect and professionalism toward its longtime partner—considerations that Planned Parenthood would not extend to Komen.

Planned Parenthood and 2012

As we were making our preliminary decisions, Planned Parenthood's rhetoric was growing more extreme in anticipation of the 2012 election cycle. In November 2011, Planned Parenthood launched WomenAreWatching.org, a militant site that is little more than a shill for the Democrats and their claim of a so-called *war on women,* a term coined by the feminist left to attack conservatives who oppose the liberal agenda, particularly on abortion. "This past year," the website said, "we have been witnessing the most aggressive legislative attacks on women's health and rights in a generation. . . . *Women Are Watching* is Planned Parenthood Action Fund's 2012 campaign to educate women across the country about the unprecedented attacks on women's health and where candidates stand on pivotal health-care issues, empower women to hold anti-women's health candidates of either party accountable, and work to elect pro-women's health candidates up and down the ballot."

The website is plastered in pink, Komen's trademark color; the color synonymous with the fight against breast cancer.

To me it was a blatant attempt by Planned Parenthood to link itself to the fight against breast cancer. Even Planned Parenthood seemed to acknowledge that abortion is highly controversial and divisive—why else were they doing so much to shift attention away from the central part of its mission? If they could somehow get people to think of them as champions for the broader cause of women's health, especially breast cancer, they could perhaps mainstream themselves. After all, the fight against breast cancer evokes compassion, not controversy.

Planned Parenthood and its political allies were hijacking the color pink, making it political and using it as a partisan baton against conservatives. Earlier in the year, Cecile Richards had inaccurately claimed that Planned Parenthood provided mammograms, and Planned Parenthood ran a series of ads that were also awash in pink.

I remember how upset Nancy was when she learned of the website. She was upset that Planned Parenthood was using the color pink, which she seemed to think could imply that Komen supported Planned Parenthood's entire agenda. It was at this point that senior management met yet again to discuss how we would proceed in 2012. There was consensus that it was imperative not to give a scalp to either side. Whatever the decision and direction forward, there could be no gaps for the women we were serving—we would lead with the mission, just as Komen always did.

The Komen board was scheduled to meet in late November. On November 20, I pointed out to Nancy that there were no easy answers and that we could not please everyone. I reiterated my genuine belief that neutral ground was the best place for Komen. I wanted Nancy to be prepared for a difficult discussion. Nancy seemed to understand what was ahead. I remember that she said Komen had no choice because being associated with something so politically charged affected our organization. Besides, she said, Planned Parenthood had created the issues, not Komen.

I was asked to provide talking points for Nancy and Liz for the November 28 board meeting and to provide briefing materials for the entire board on the matter. I reinforced that the new criteria were not aimed at Planned Parenthood specifically—they were much broader, and Planned Parenthood was just one of various grantees we expected to be affected by these higher performance standards and stricter criteria. We were not terminating any of Planned Parenthood's grants. However, Planned Parenthood would be ineligible for grants as of January 1, 2012—based on our more stringent granting criteria. Further, while Planned

Parenthood would not be barred from applying indefinitely, the types of programs they offer would not meet the new outcomes-based standards. Investigations—not simply the one launched by the congressional committee—were just *one* of the many issues that brought us to this place.

As I pointed out earlier, had Komen been enforcing its existing criteria, Planned Parenthood would have already been deemed ineligible and the existing grants revoked. Komen had to have the ability to protect its mission and the organization in the event that *any* organization with which we were partnered (whether through grants, marketing, etc.) had challenges or issues that were so serious that Komen was negatively affected. Unfortunately, with regards to Planned Parenthood, that was where Komen found itself.

To my surprise, the board meeting went smoothly—very smoothly. Several board members asked questions. However, not a single one raised concerns about or objected to moving forward with the strategy and supporting criteria as of January 1.

Internal Commotion

Liz wanted to personally tell Mollie Williams face-to-face about the decision before we moved ahead. I respected that Liz was handling the situation this way.

After the meeting, Liz came down to my office—I happened to be in Dallas that day—to tell me about it.

The media reported that Mollie resigned over the decision. I suppose that was partly true. The media also reported that the resignation was immediate. That was not true. Certainly I appreciated Mollie's disappointment, but I believed that Mollie's decision was based on far more than the decision regarding the grants program and its effect on Planned Parenthood. I suspected that the Planned Parenthood decision was her last straw. Komen had recently launched a search for a community health vice president to oversee the entire community grants program.

Also, one has to keep in mind that the new granting standards were going into effect one way or another, sooner or later. This was a case of sooner. And Mollie had to know, based on Liz's numerous comments about limiting education and pass-through grants, that Planned Parenthood would be affected. I wondered if Mollie would have spilled a single tear for the other organizations that would be affected. It seemed to me that, like various affiliate employees in the summer meeting, Mollie may have been struggling to balance her loyalty to Komen with her support of Planned Parenthood and their pro-choice mission.

I had no idea that Mollie's emotional reaction would pale in comparison to the cries of the left.

The Infiltration

I headed into December thinking that everyone was on the same page. What I did not know was that there were those within who had divided loyalties between Komen and Planned Parenthood. And—what was worse—we had invited them into our ranks.

Komen had several public relations firms on retainer. Morris

+ King in New York. Ogilvy in Washington, D.C.—our account rep there was Brendan Daly. I didn't work with him directly; in fact, I met him in person for the first time during the week of the firestorm. Most of his interaction was with Leslie in communications or directly with Nancy, who often bypassed staff to talk with consultants directly.

Ari Fleischer had so far been unsuccessful in finding a viable candidate to lead the communications role at Komen. Leslie continued in her role. Brendan was brought up to speed on the decision and its effect on Planned Parenthood. He and Leslie were to work through various scenarios and communications issues.

I would later learn that Brendan Daly had been the communications director to House Minority Leader Nancy Pelosi. He and Cecile Richards had worked together in Pelosi's office. Yep, *that* Cecile Richards, who is now the CEO of Planned Parenthood.

Sometime in November, a new PR gal was hired to supplement the consultants Komen already had on retainer. She was with a firm called SKDKnickerbocker. Her name was Hilary Rosen.

Rosen was an ardent liberal, outspoken gay rights advocate, and combative talking head on the Sunday morning political shows. I doubt anyone at Komen knew she was also working for the Democratic National Committee (DNC), providing media training to its new head, Congresswoman Debbie Wasserman Schultz. During the 2012 election cycle, the DNC has so far paid Rosen's firm as a "communications consultant" and as a "media consultant," with SKDKnickerbocker raking in more than $120,000.[8] Rosen was meeting regularly with the White House.[9] Rosen's partner at SKDKnickerbocker was former Obama head of communications Anita Dunn. SKDKnickerbocker also served as Sandra Fluke's publicist during the Rush Limbaugh controversy.

Later, Rosen would become famous for suggesting that Mitt Romney's wife, Ann, hadn't worked "a day in her life."

But for Komen, she was just somebody who was hired to help us navigate the treacherous waters of Planned Parenthood and the related sea of politics. Liz and Nancy wanted someone to manage the left, and I certainly wasn't the right person for that.

Nancy and Liz hired Rosen directly. As far as I know, no one else at Komen had any interactions with her before she was brought on board. Liz announced the hiring of Rosen, informing us that Rosen's job was to create appropriate messaging for what Liz called the fringe groups. Rosen and her team apparently had specific strategies in mind for how to best communicate to this constituency. Rosen and her SKDKnickerbocker associates would manage the left on issues such as the Promise Me perfume, possible environmental causes for breast cancer—and Planned Parenthood.

Liz introduced Rosen to me as Komen's Planned Parenthood point person. I would manage the issue on the right and ensure appropriate coordination within Komen, while Hilary would manage the left and be our liaison with Planned Parenthood. I have no idea how I was described to Hilary, but I think she may have been told that I was Komen's point person on the right—as

I was told Hilary would be the point person on the left. I think this is probably where the leftist strategy began to be formulated in which the entire Planned Parenthood issue would be dumped in my lap.

Right after Hilary's introduction, Leslie came to me with disturbing news. She wanted to know if I was familiar with Hilary. I was not, but Leslie seemed to be and described Hilary as a heavy-hitter Democrat in D.C. Leslie also told me that she thought Hilary's firm was also Planned Parenthood's PR firm. In response to Liz's introductory email, Hilary had responded that her colleague Emily Lenzner was her firm's "Planned Parenthood expert."

It would later turn out that Leslie's initial thought about SKDKnickerbocker and Planned Parenthood was right. Leslie and I discussed on numerous occasions whether this was a conflict. Leslie raised the issue with Liz directly. I weighed in as well, having multiple conversations with both Liz and Nancy. I pushed my concerns about as far as I thought I could. Nonetheless, Rosen was hired. And, in one discussion with Hilary, I specifically raised my concerns that SKDKnickerbocker was representing both Komen and Planned Parenthood. Hilary reassured us by saying that there was a "firewall between their clients," so we had nothing to be concerned about.

Rosen brought with her the expertise of Emily Lenzner, who was to help us manage media relations. Rosen again described her as their firm's Planned Parenthood expert. Did it mean that Emily worked directly with Planned Parenthood? If so, I worried even more about this individual being a key member of Komen's team. Lenzner had been the executive director of communications for ABC News in Washington, where she handled publicity for George Stephanopoulos, Christiane Amanpour, Jake Tapper, and Ted Koppel. Her husband, Peter Cherukuri, was general manager of the D.C. bureau of the *Huffington Post*. The connection to the *Huffington Post* would later seem to be another happenstance in a growing list of coincidences. The *Huffington Post* would become the media outlet of choice for various supposed Komen insiders, generally anonymous, who were aiding the left in pushing the lie that I had somehow single-handedly convinced Komen to transition out of the Planned Parenthood grants.

Komen did not view Planned Parenthood as our enemy—or even a potential enemy. Our hired experts—Hilary Rosen and SKDKnickerbocker—never portrayed Planned Parenthood as our enemy. But I should have known better. I should have pushed even harder about what I saw as a gross conflict of interest. Given my political background, I should have anticipated the fury of the liberals—this was about Planned Parenthood, the icon of the left. I also should have trusted my instincts that Planned Parenthood could not be trusted. I also went to such lengths to keep politics out of our decision and our approach that I failed to anticipate the political firestorm that would await us. I can only say that I believed the counsel and feedback we were receiving from Rosen were accurate and sound—and I believed that those around me did as well.

Komen and Planned Parenthood were longtime friends who were simply going to have to go in different directions. Komen wanted to do so amicably and we did our best to achieve this. Planned Parenthood, however, attempted to destroy Komen, quite literally, for what I believe had everything to do with politics and nothing to do with the grants themselves. Ari Fleischer would later remark that Komen was simply no match for Planned Parenthood. That was certainly true, but in my view, it seemed as though Planned Parenthood benefited from the misreads and incorrect assessments of Komen's very own consultants, including Hilary Rosen, who had assured and reassured us time and again.

Call it naïveté. Call it stupidity. Incompetence. Wishful thinking. But for our part, we were genuinely committed to avoiding a media firestorm for ourselves and for Planned Parenthood. And we believed that Planned Parenthood shared this desire.

Planned Parenthood would not share this commitment, and Komen would soon find itself at the business end of a knife, one wielded by an irate ex-partner who would stop at nothing to keep us together.

5

A Gentle-ladies' Agreement

It was now the beginning of December. Legal and community health were revising the grant criteria and related documents for rolling out the new granting strategy. Leslie was developing the press statements in case we needed them. We had to advise the entire affiliate network. Because of Komen's long friendship with Planned Parenthood and Hilary's counsel, everyone remained hopeful that an amicable break—a gentle-ladies' agreement, if you will, would be reached.

Hilary Rosen was pushing hard for a conference call with Cecile Richards of Planned Parenthood. Liz considered Cecile a friend, and I sensed that she felt an obligation to talk directly to Cecile.

I was wary. To me, the solution seemed simple: roll out the new granting strategy and revised criteria and proceed as we normally would through the application and selection process. The affiliate granting cycles were staggered throughout the year. Organizations, including Planned Parenthood, would either meet the new standards or they would not. We were not doing pre-calls to any other grantees that might be affected, so singling out Planned Parenthood did not seem to be a prudent approach. With that said, I also knew that it was important for our affiliates to be advised of the changes before they heard it from somewhere else. I was concerned that, once Liz talked to Cecile, Planned Parenthood would begin putting pressure on our affiliates.

The Scramble

The first week of December was a scramble. Internal Q&A documents were developed for our affiliates. I understood the need to give them as much information and guidance as possible, but I was concerned that the document was far too detailed and emphasized Planned Parenthood far too much.

Given Komen National's sometimes strained relationship with the affiliates, we went above and beyond to be transparent and provide as much information to them as possible. A call with the affiliates that had active Planned Parenthood grants was held on December 6. In retrospect, this was a bad idea. Our intent was to reach out to these affiliates first. Other grantees would be affected, but Planned Parenthood was the only grantee that was a national network with multiple grants across the country. We knew that some in the affiliate ranks would not be agreeable because of the impact on Planned Parenthood. Liz gave an overview of outcomes-based granting. This was more of a review for the affiliates, because Komen's move to this new strategy was not new; it had been under way since 2010. Liz explained that this was the first in what would be several rounds of changes in the coming year, as we fully implemented the outcomes-based grant strategy, and that these stricter criteria supported our new granting direction. Liz walked through the new criteria, including the more stringent language regarding financial and administrative improprieties and investigations. Our donors expected us to have the highest standards—for ourselves, our grants, and our grantees. She underscored our commitment to ensuring no gaps for the women we served. The response was a mix of relief and anger. Many of the affiliates on the call came across as comforted to know that this difficult, time-consuming issue would finally be off their plate. Others objected vehemently in what seemed like an overly emotional response—more in support of Planned Parenthood than Komen.

Liz would convey a similar assessment to Nancy, noting the range of reactions. I agreed and pointed out that some appeared to overreact, focused more on Planned Parenthood's best interest than ours, especially since the individual grants to Planned Parenthood were generally a very small percentage of any one affiliate's total community grant portfolio. I doubted these same affiliates would be as upset about any other organizations.

Earlier that week, Komen's PR consultant Brendan Daly, from Ogilvy, was brought into the loop. He proposed a statement for possible press use. To my dismay, what he provided focused on the stricter criteria and that Komen was exercising its option to terminate future grants to Planned Parenthood.

I wasn't Komen's communications lead, but this struck me as terrible. First, we were not terminating any of the grants. Second,

I continued to have concerns about any public statement that focused specifically on Planned Parenthood. Third, with or without
investigations, Planned Parenthood's grants were largely educational in nature and pass-through grants—the very type of grants
we were moving away from. Liz's reaction was that the proposed
statement was not good.

On December 6, Leslie and Brendan discussed the situation.
They provided an overview of their thoughts and recommendations regarding potential communications scenarios. It was in
this overview that I first learned of Brendan's connection to Cecile Richards. I knew that he had previously worked for Pelosi,
but it was news to me that, during his tenure in Pelosi's office,
Cecile was his colleague. According to Leslie, Brendan knew
Cecile well. Various scenarios that Planned Parenthood might
pursue if they decided to go public included bombarding Komen
with emails and calls, asking various women's organizations to
stop supporting Komen, and asking Komen friends in Congress,
including Debbie Wasserman Schultz, to pressure Komen. Leslie
and Brendan also said we could likely expect petitions and negative coverage from various blogs, publications, and social media.

The scenario turned out to be right on target. Daly had worked
with Cecile at Pelosi's office, and his resume trumpets him as
a Democratic strategist. I did not make that connection, and it
would later be another concern—and yet another coincidence.

Looking back, I wonder at the many coincidences. Here was
another link between Komen's consultants and the organiza-

tion that would soon become our adversary and try to destroy us. Today, I have a lot of questions. Was Brendan in contact with Cecile? With the Democratic Party? Were the personal politics of our consultants and even some Komen employees taking priority over Komen's best interests? Much was made about me being a conservative and that my personal views drove the decision within Komen—which was not true. But if my personal beliefs were fair game, why weren't those who had views on the other side of the aisle subjected to the same scrutiny?

Over the next few days, Leslie and her team, presumably with Brendan, continued to work through the media messaging. Liz, Katrina, legal, community health, and I weighed in on the numerous iterations of the document. Finally, it seemed that we had settled on an approach that everyone seemed to agree with—or at least mostly agreed with. We would conduct no proactive media outreach—granting strategies and criteria changed with relative frequency, affecting various organizations along the way, and we would keep our commitment to Planned Parenthood. Our statement to have "on the ready" would focus on maintaining the highest degree of integrity with our grants and on the new granting strategy and stricter criteria that would enable us to do so; that women we served remained our highest priority. With this, I agreed.

But the statement still had the sentence singling out Planned Parenthood. Liz also seemed concerned about this. Why were we identifying Planned Parenthood specifically rather than simply saying these criteria determine eligibility in applying for a grant?

But Leslie argued that, if the press called, it would be specific to Planned Parenthood. I supposed that was true, but I still thought it was a mistake to get into a detailed exchange over the finer details and to foster a focus on Planned Parenthood. Keep it simple: "We have a new granting strategy and more stringent criteria going forward. Various grants and grantees will be affected. This will allow Komen to do more for the women we serve and do it more effectively." Anything more seemed defensive—after all, Komen had a right to establish whatever granting strategy and criteria it believed was best for the organization; no apologies were needed.

Hilary Rosen was to provide input—Nancy and Liz directed. To me it seemed as though we were going in circles—round and round. With so many consultants, advice was conflicting.

About this time, I made my own serious miscalculation—related to the political reaction. I didn't think members of Congress would make an issue out of Komen's decision—as long as we focused on our granting policy. I figured that Cecile would go to her friends in the Democratic leadership, but I believed that Wasserman Schultz, as head of the DNC, and others were focused on bigger things. I could not have been more wrong. I did not anticipate that the passion and support for Planned Parenthood would make Komen expendable; that Komen would be seen as necessary collateral damage. I also failed to see the converging issues of contraception, women's health, and the 2012 elections, and that Komen would be swept up in the "war on women."

Hilary offered her version of a standby press statement. Again I thought there was too much focus on Planned Parenthood and investigations. I felt that making the investigations criteria the focal point of anything we said publicly would give Planned Parenthood an excuse to claim that we were targeting them for political reasons. I thought Liz agreed.

But on December 7, Rosen provided her suggested version of a press statement. It contained specific language that Planned Parenthood was facing the kind of ongoing investigations that are covered in the new criteria and that the organization would be ineligible for new funding until the investigations were complete. Her proposed statement noted that Komen was making no assertions of any improprieties, and Liz would later tell me that Hilary recommended warmer statements of mutual respect.

I remained concerned. First, investigations or not, it was my understanding that the new strategy would generally preclude the types of grants we funded with Planned Parenthood and others. Further, I didn't think we could finalize anything until Liz spoke with Cecile and we had the benefit of her reaction. Nevertheless, this language would serve as the foundation for much of our communications going forward. We would play right into Planned Parenthood's hands.

The Leak

On December 8, from a hotel conference room in San Antonio where many of us from Komen were attending the annual San

Antonio Breast Cancer Symposium, I participated in a conference call with Liz, Nancy, and Hilary Rosen.

Hilary gave us her rationale for the proposed statement she had provided the day before. She seemed hypersensitive about Komen saying anything that could be interpreted as negative about Planned Parenthood's work. This was curious to me— hadn't Komen already come to the conclusion that these grants would not meet our standards? I didn't see it as negative toward Planned Parenthood that Komen was changing its granting direction, but I agreed with being as magnanimous as possible.

The crucial point conveyed on the call, though, was Hilary's risk assessment. She told us that she believed Planned Parenthood had bigger fish to fry than to pick a fight with an organization as trusted and loved as Komen. She advised that once Liz talked with Cecile, the two organizations could work through things. Hilary's assessment of Planned Parenthood's reaction was met with what I think was relief all around. Nancy and Liz had said that Hilary was hired because she was wired into Cecile and the left, so I believe we all thought we were getting sound counsel and accurate intel.

While the back-and-forth continued on the press-related materials, the same process was under way with materials for the affiliates. A detailed Q&A document, addressing every imaginable scenario and question that might be raised, was developed. This document contained the question "On what basis is Planned Parenthood no longer eligible to receive Komen grants?" And it would be this question that Planned Parenthood would later put in our face.

The answer focused entirely on the stricter eligibility criteria—and the investigations. This was technically correct, but also somewhat incomplete. The response failed to provide the more fundamental reason for the change—that we were moving away from the types of grants Planned Parenthood offered; doing away with poor-quality grants. And the response did not address our broader concerns about the impact of Planned Parenthood's controversies on our organization and how these issues were indeed *a* part of our decision. All of this was addressed elsewhere, but this would not stop Planned Parenthood from singling out this one question and our answer to make its case against us.

You might be wondering why the affiliate document had questions specific to Planned Parenthood in the first place. In hindsight, perhaps it shouldn't have. The criteria affected all organizations. As we rolled out the new granting approach, education grants would significantly decline and we would move away from pass-through grants where possible. This would affect many organizations, not just Planned Parenthood. As we developed the stricter eligibility and performance standards to support the new granting model, we already knew of one other organization that would be affected: the indigent care hospital in a major metropolitan city; and we expected others. But Planned Parenthood would be the most affected. Planned Parenthood as a whole received from fifteen to twenty grants in any given year. We should have also made it crystal clear that the congressional investigation, while a concern, was not the driving factor.

To our own detriment, this document was created and distributed widely to Komen's affiliate network—and quickly made its way into the hands of Planned Parenthood.

Rosen was now firmly established as Komen's go-to liaison with Planned Parenthood. Liz relied on Rosen for counsel on how to handle her call with Cecile and would refer to Rosen as "our friend." Months later, I would wonder if Hilary really was our friend.

Rosen facilitated a call between Liz and Cecile, but Cecile did not answer at the scheduled time. Liz continued calling Cecile for days.

Meanwhile, word was out. On December 15, one of Komen's founding board members, also a major Planned Parenthood ally, contacted Nancy. She told Nancy that she had been contacted by the head of a local Planned Parenthood chapter who told her about a rumor circulating that related to Komen—that the Komen board had voted to defund Planned Parenthood because someone in Washington was investigating. The former Komen board member wanted Nancy to meet with Cecile Richards and Planned Parenthood's board chair, Cecilia Boone.

That wasn't the only indication that there was a leak. One of our Komen affiliates contacted us. Apparently the local Planned Parenthood chapter had contacted the Komen affiliate to say that Planned Parenthood higher-ups were in a room discussing information that the Komen board was about to vote to block all grants. The Planned Parenthood person said the decision was supposedly driven by a particular Komen board member and asked if there was a way to broker a conversation between Liz and Cecile in order to avoid a tragic situation for women.

My guess is that the Komen board member that Planned Parenthood was apparently blaming was Jane Abraham. Jane was on Komen's board, and she was also board president of the pro-life organization Susan B. Anthony List. It was not true that any of this had been at her direction or doing.

I certainly had not anticipated that someone within Komen would leak information to Planned Parenthood. And the information had to have been leaked, because none of the information had been distributed publicly. In fact, we had not yet even distributed the affiliate Q&A document across the affiliate network. I can say that I was deeply disturbed that anyone who was part of the Komen family would do this. But as I would point out to everyone, it was done, and now we needed to ensure that our internal team was briefed. Liz seemed as agitated about the leak as I was. However, no action was taken, and leaks would continue in the coming weeks.

That same night, Liz drafted an email to Cecile. She appeared to want to make the first move, seemingly bothered that Cecile was already generating calls to Nancy. Her note was an explanation of our new grants approach and the impact on Planned Parenthood, and it reflected Hilary's linguistic suggestions. I was under the impression that Hilary was coordinating all communication with Cecile, and I think Nancy and everyone else thought this, as well. At this point, Katrina McGhee, Komen's executive vice president of marketing, weighed in. She cautioned about being overly effusive in writing and suggested that a short, to-the-point, compassionate note followed by a personal conversation was a better approach. Liz responded that her draft email included wording from Hilary and reiterated that the press statement, if needed, had come from Hilary. I thought the implication of Liz's comments was obvious: we would rely on Hilary's counsel.

Nancy seemed to already be getting anxious, after just one email, and asked about a backup plan should Cecile come out swinging. She seemed concerned that the fire had already been lit.

Of course, there could be no "Plan B" in terms of the Planned Parenthood grants. We could not be half pregnant—Planned Parenthood either met the new criteria or it did not. We had decided it did not, based on our new grant strategy and criteria. Cecile would be mad. And she might well go on the attack—boycotting Komen races just as the pro-lifers were doing. We were prepared for that—expecting that. Leslie and Brendan were preparing the contingency plan. We had discussed on numerous occasions the risks—and rewards—of the direction we were pursuing, including that there would likely be a short-term hit to Komen, including a dip in fund-raising, as we shifted to neutral ground. But still, we believed that being on neutral ground was the stronger ground.

Meanwhile, the backlash and PR issues continued as a backdrop. The pink Bible issue generated tremendous media coverage with stories on CNN and in the *New York Times,* along with virtually every TV and print outlet in the country. At the same time, the State of Wisconsin would be the next state to strip funding from Planned Parenthood. And so the steady drip, drip, drip continued.

Finally, on December 16, Liz and Cecile connected.

Liz and Cecile spoke one-on-one—or least no one from Komen was with Liz. Liz related that Cecile reacted with a range of emotions—from sounding as though she was crying to seeming angry. But by the end of the call, Liz believed that she and Cecile had agreed that it was in no one's interest to create a firestorm. They agreed to a follow-up call the next week—with others from Planned Parenthood and Komen.

Liz also wrote to Hilary to fill her in on the call. I now wonder if Hilary wasn't already up to speed. Liz and I spoke that night after her call with Cecile and again numerous times over the weekend. Liz said that Cecile was emotional and insisted that the issue would be media fodder, but Liz reassured her that no one at Komen wanted that to happen. Liz said that they discussed how each organization would respond. Liz underscored that Komen would not discuss the issue in the press, but she said Cecile insisted that she would have to respond and go on the attack. Liz said she prevailed on Cecile to consider that antagonism between the two organizations would not be in the best interest of the women we both served and our shared donors. Liz also said Cecile noted in their call that she already knew exactly what was coming, and this internal betrayal seemed to anger Liz greatly. Yet, Liz conveyed that she was optimistic; that it was natural for Cecile to have this initial reaction and, over the weekend, Cecile would have a chance to calm down.

Liz also gave additional direction to Hilary. She said she wanted Hilary to reach out to Cecile and work with her. Good, I thought. That was, after all, why Hilary was hired. Liz also made it clear that, if Planned Parenthood took an aggressive stance, Komen would have to take a stronger approach.

Hilary responded that, no matter what Planned Parenthood did, Komen must not take the bait. She advised that we respond with the statement and make sure we praise Planned Parenthood's work, as a way to endear ourselves to the media and the public.

I agreed we should not take the bait. We needed to stay professional and aboveboard. But if Planned Parenthood launched an all-out assault, I didn't see how endorsing the work of our assaulters was the appropriate way to respond for Komen. Komen would also decline to take an aggressive stance when Planned Parenthood attacked, choosing instead to surrender.

The Escalation

That night, after her conversation with Cecile, Liz sent a follow-up email, telling Cecile that she hoped the organizations could keep the situation from escalating in the media and with donors. Liz provided Cecile with Komen's top-line messaging, which by now had been revised to make no mention whatsoever of investigations.

The next morning, we heard from Cecile directly. She was apparently angry that Komen had sent information about the grants policy to our affiliates before contacting her. To me, her position was completely unreasonable. We had to communicate internally—the affiliates were part of *our organization*. And we hadn't sent anything to the press. Nonetheless, Cecile used our internal document as a club to beat us. She specifically characterized the decision as political and said that our ability to manage any fallout from the decision was compromised when Komen chose to communicate directly with its affiliates before allowing Planned Parenthood to review the materials.

Again, I thought this was an irrational and ridiculous demand. First, these were internal documents and policies. Komen had no obligation to include Cecile in our review process, and it was unreasonable to expect that. It seemed to me that Cecile was trying to find a way to blame Komen for how she was going to respond. She specifically used the word *fallout*. What fallout? There would only be fallout if Planned Parenthood went to war. We were working with her—out of professional courtesy and respect. We weren't obligated to do so; we chose to.

Although I would not recognize it then—and no one else seemed to either—Cecile had just thrown down her marker. Komen's decision would be portrayed as politics. Still, Komen had given its word—which we would keep—that we would not go to the press. And, as conversations and email exchanges continued between our two organizations, it was our belief that we were still working toward a mutually agreeable resolution.

Looking back, it is now clear to me that Cecile telegraphed her playbook in her note. But, I believe, in being so focused on how to shield Planned Parenthood from any negative reaction, Komen failed to recognize Planned Parenthood as even a potential enemy. I don't believe anyone seriously thought that Planned Parenthood would literally try to destroy Komen. We were too busy worrying about how to minimize Planned Parenthood's hurt feelings—instead of focusing on our mission and a decision that was made to best support that mission. I think we would all come to regret this.

It was Saturday. It would be a long weekend. I took some time to put together my initial thoughts on a worst-case scenario should we not reach consensus and Planned Parenthood go nuclear. I wanted to relay my thoughts to everyone first thing on Monday. My scenario included Cecile hitting the airwaves and blasting Komen. I still believed that our response should take the high road, regardless of the path Planned Parenthood chose. We could acknowledge Planned Parenthood's disappointment but should emphasize that we were focused on our mission, that we respected Planned Parenthood's need to do what was necessary for its mission, and that we had hoped they would respect our need to do the same for ours; their actions were disappointing. I continued to see a simple statement focused on our mission as the best approach rather than allowing ourselves to get mired in the details and complexities of the granting process.

On Monday I was on the Planned Parenthood call with Liz. Several people from Planned Parenthood were on the call, including Dawn Laguens, executive vice president for policy, advocacy, and communications.

Oddly, Hilary Rosen was not on the call. I thought it was strange, because this is the kind of call that I thought Liz would have wanted Hilary to be a part of. If she was our consultant to "manage the left" and our Planned Parenthood liaison, shouldn't she have been on the call?

Let me stop for a minute to highlight yet another link that I discovered between Komen's consultants and Planned Parenthood. Hilary and Dawn were clearly acquainted. They had a connection through the same small private school in Washington, D.C. The coincidences just kept piling up.

The call with Planned Parenthood was the first time I should have realized that I would personally end up the number-one target for Planned Parenthood's hit squad. Here's why. Dawn or someone on the call from Planned Parenthood addressed me personally: "We've done a little research on you, Karen. We've read your writings on Planned Parenthood."

The comment took me aback. Writings? I didn't have any "writings" on Planned Parenthood. There was a blurb about my pro-life beliefs on the website for my governor's campaign. I'm sure it mentioned Planned Parenthood, but that was it. Annoyed but chuckling a bit at the irony, I replied, "If you'd really done your homework on me, you would know that I'm not some darling of the pro-life moment. Second, I'm a professional, and I don't appreciate the comment that this has something to do with my politics. Komen has people of every political belief; but when we come to Komen, we are all here for one thing: to fight breast cancer."

Liz, too, seemed annoyed by the personal attack.

Then we got down to specifics. We reiterated that we were not "defunding" any grants and confirmed that we would pay out all current grants. We also advised that four grants, totaling approximately $200,000, would continue for at least another grant cycle.

The discussion was not without further rancor. Liz reviewed our new grant strategy and the stricter criteria. Specifically, Liz mentioned the criteria regarding an organization being barred from government funding. This provoked vehement denials from the Planned Parenthood side, that this was not true. Except that it was true. They argued the reasons for the loss of state funding—blaming ideology, politics, and even saying that they had "lost" funding but weren't "barred" from applying. None of this was our concern. The contract language was what it was. And, remember, this contract requirement was not new—it had been part of the Komen grant contracts all along. And Planned Parenthood had been signing these contracts year after year. Nevertheless, we reassured Planned Parenthood that we would rework all existing contracts to ensure full payout of current grants.

The conversation ended on what seemed to be a calmer and encouraging note. Both organizations agreed to exchange statements and work together on messaging. There was a mutual understanding that we would not go to the press proactively, and if something changed, we would not blindside one another. I believed progress had been made, and Liz seemed to think so, too.

By this time, our first-line media statement had changed more times than I could count. Finally, though, we had a statement that focused on three key points: our mission, the women we serve, and a new granting model that would strengthen our community impact. Not investigations.

Meanwhile, more leaks. The following day, December 19, before we had even had a chance to send over the proposed statement, Dawn emailed us. She was focused on something else altogether—the internal Q&A document that had been provided to our affiliates earlier. How did Planned Parenthood have this document? It had been distributed internally, with only the Komen Board, leadership team, affiliates—and Komen's PR consultants—receiving it. Once again, someone from the Komen family had to have leaked the information to Planned Parenthood. Dawn zeroed in on two specific questions—the answers to which were drawn from Hilary's earlier suggested statement. Dawn said that the responses did not reflect Komen's message of shifting grant strategies.

I thought we should get ready for combat. It seemed to me that Planned Parenthood was simply stringing us along and looking for a pretext to declare war. But Hilary continued to advise that we not take the bait, that it was a positive sign that we were still going back and forth, and no one from Planned Parenthood indicated that we had reached an impasse. So we continued to work on a mutually agreeable message.

On December 20, Liz emailed Cecile with the proposed statement. She thanked Cecile for her patience as the organizations worked through the issues together. She reiterated that we had not and would not contact any media. It was a friendly email and underscored our continued desire to work cooperatively with Planned Parenthood.

Dawn, rather than Cecile, responded. She made several suggestions about how to answer any questions specific to Planned Parenthood. She also requested that we recall the information we had provided to our affiliates for internal use.

On December 21, John Raffaelli, a Democratic lobbyist who serves on Komen's board and had indicated to me and others that he was close with Planned Parenthood, informed us that he had spoken to a top executive at Planned Parenthood that he knew. Based on his conversation, he said it was his sense that Planned Parenthood would work with us. Liz seemed understandably pleased with this news.

It seemed that things were cooling down—perhaps Hilary was right. Maybe Planned Parenthood would act with us instead of against us.

As Christmas approached, the board was given a full update on where things stood. Liz expressed her optimism that we could work through the situation without it escalating to the media and that communications with the leadership at Planned Parenthood was ongoing. She also thanked Raffaelli for his assistance with Planned Parenthood.

Shortly after the update, we began receiving phone calls from influential donors and longtime supporters from across the country who supported Komen and Planned Parenthood. We talked through the situation with them, explaining the rationale behind the decision and answering their questions. In virtually every instance, these individuals were reassured; their concerns resolved.

The Warning Shot

A few days before Christmas, we received a letter from Cecile Richards requesting a meeting with our entire Board of Directors. It was unprecedented for any grantee to meet with the full board about a grant request. Komen gave thousands of community and research grants each year, and thousands more were rejected. It was apparent to me that no one wanted to begin the practice of allowing audiences with the board over specific grant requests.

I remember one point in Cecile's letter that struck me particularly. Planned Parenthood noted that it had never been barred from receiving government funding "for any reason related to wrongdoing." The letter said that we claimed wrongdoing by Planned Parenthood in our materials.

We never said that there was wrongdoing. I was beginning to connect the dots. This was the same nuanced language that Planned Parenthood had used in our phone call. It seemed deceptive. Planned Parenthood had indeed been barred from government funding at the state level. I guess Planned Parenthood had to add the qualifier of "wrongdoing" in order to make its case. What they did not seem to grasp is that Komen's contracts allowed for no qualifiers. The rationale for debarment was not a factor.

Beyond that, the investigations weren't the only reason for ending the grants to Planned Parenthood. They were *one* reason—and a reason that seemed to have been overemphasized by Rosen and other Planned Parenthood allies within our organization. To be sure, the criteria regarding investigations affected Planned Parenthood, but the quality of its grants and the fact that Komen was going to demand much higher performance standards affected Planned Parenthood at least as much—if not more. It seemed to me that some within Komen just didn't want to admit that the grants to Planned Parenthood were low quality and that our resources could be put to better use. It seemed that some just wanted to grant to Planned Parenthood— out of loyalty to it or because that's what Komen has always done.

I could see where Planned Parenthood was going with this request. They wanted an audience with the board and would try to enflame our board members—several of whom I thought were strong supporters of Planned Parenthood.

I thought the letter was incredibly audacious. In it, Cecile said that Planned Parenthood was a leader in breast health and cancer detection. By whose standards? Planned Parenthood was a leader in a number of things, but I don't think that most reasonable people would identify Planned Parenthood as a leader in breast health or cancer detection. Planned Parenthood said Komen's action were political and said that we had based our decision on politically motivated investigations where there was no proof of malfeasance. It was interesting to me that Planned Parenthood failed to reference any of the improprieties that had been proven over the years.

The letter took aim at the investigations issue and made the case that the internal document provided to the Komen affiliates contained misleading information and that this misinformation was already shaping the public narrative.

There was no public narrative—at least not yet. In fact, we did not want a public narrative at all. We had no intention of ever making "investigations" the public narrative or mentioning it with the press, and we told Planned Parenthood that repeatedly. Unfortunately, someone would eventually do so—Komen's own communications vice president, Leslie Aun.

We should have seen the letter for what it was—a foreshadowing of things to come. Planned Parenthood would play the victim, accusing Komen of being bullies and succumbing to political pressure—despite the fact that they were actually in breach of the existing contracts.

Making themselves the victims was ingenious on Planned Parenthood's part. Komen indeed wanted an exit strategy from Planned Parenthood. But Komen always kept its mission and the women we served first and foremost in our deliberations, and the decision to disengage from Planned Parenthood was a reasonable one made with women and our mission as the priority.

I thought that Planned Parenthood was making a much bigger issue of this than $680,000 in annual grants seemed to warrant. Why? Losing this funding would have virtually no impact given its sizable budget. We would soon find out the reason.

I told Liz and Nancy that the letter felt like a setup. I do not believe in coincidences and there were just way too many. I felt strongly that we had to avoid getting into a back-and-forth on each issue. It seemed to me that Planned Parenthood was laying out its talking points. They would say that Komen made the decision largely because of investigations; that they tried to work it out with us, but we refused their suggestions and requests; that they had no choice—women were at risk.

Nancy responded to me that Komen had to serve its mission—regardless of consequences. She stressed her belief that we had to measure our work. It seemed to me that Nancy was reiterating her commitment to moving forward. We would deal with whatever came our way—because what we were doing did, indeed, best serve our mission.

The Christmas break was here, and we let Planned Parenthood know that Komen would close down until after New Year's Day. We would respond after the Christmas break to the letter requesting a meeting with the board.

As we headed off for Christmas, Komen was still negotiating with Planned Parenthood, and we believed that Planned Parenthood was in the same posture. But I worried about what would happen if we refused one of Planned Parenthood's demands. Would they go to war? My angst over whether Komen really had the "stomach for a fight" was growing—as I recalled that general assessment of Komen from my very first meeting with Komen about the consulting work.

I should have followed my gut and sounded the alarm. Instead I worried about being called "political" and biased for thinking the worst of Planned Parenthood.

Over Christmas, the stress of it all finally caught up with me. I am not easily brought to tears. I'd been on my own since age seventeen. I am tough. I'd been through the heartbreak of not being able to have a child. Pro-life bullies called me desperate and barren, because in their view I wasn't quite pro-life enough. I told Steve, tears in my eyes, "I hate this. I came to Komen to get away from this."

The pro-life issue just kept resurfacing as a central theme in my life. I talked to one of my close friends about it. "You'll do your best," she told me. "But I've gotta tell you, you need to do some praying about this, girlfriend, because you're always in the middle of it."

To be sure, I had my own feelings about Planned Parenthood and abortion, but I also had a job to do and that meant keeping my politics and personal views separate. When I joined Komen, I disengaged from anything political—except voting, of course. That fall, I even turned down a tremendous opportunity to join the board of the Republican State Leadership Committee, chaired at the time by Ed Gillespie. On anything related to the Republican presidential primary, I passed. I was committed to Komen, to our mission, and I was not going to do anything that would limit my effectiveness.

I could not shake the terrible sense of dread. I felt in my heart of hearts that Komen would not have the fortitude to see this through. I knew that there were those who sided with Planned Parenthood—even to Komen's detriment.

My concerns were magnified by other issues, too. Nancy and Liz seemed steadfast one day and unsure the next. If they weren't 100 percent certain, if they had any doubts, we should not move forward. With so many consultants, we were getting conflicting advice. Complicated issues that required serious discussion were too often relegated to a multitude of email exchanges.

In being directed to coordinate this project, I felt like I had been asked to conduct an orchestra—to develop a public policy strategy and help coordinate a PR strategy. I was supposed to deliver a soaring symphony—yet the strings section failed to show, the woodwinds brought their own sheet music, and the brass refused to play. I was trying to deliver on a project when I felt I didn't have the support and internal buy-in required for success. I was trying to do a job with leadership that seemed sometimes uncertain about taking a stand, a communications function in flux, and outside PR counsel that I questioned. I was already the odd gal out at Komen. I was the "righty tighty," and I knew some saw me as the instigator about Planned Parenthood. I knew about the claims that I was exaggerating the Planned Parenthood backlash.

And so I found myself wasting precious time during the Christmas break, stressing and obsessing about it all instead of enjoying my time with Steve and family. I wondered. Komen said it wanted out of the Planned Parenthood grants, but did they really? Would they really see it through? I was having serious doubts. I sensed a disaster in the making—and somehow knew that I would be the scapegoat.

The Calm Before the Storm

Over the Christmas break, I reflected on that last Planned Parenthood missive. It was incredible. It was filled with factual errors. It said we should have reached out to them before we communicated to our own team. It said that we were shifting from prevention and screening of breast cancer to research funding. That wasn't true, especially because there is no such thing as breast cancer prevention. Planned Parenthood claimed to be a major cancer organization. That, too, was a ridiculous claim. Planned Parenthood is a reproductive and sexual health organization and a powerful political organization spending millions of dollars as an agent of the Democratic Party.

I drafted a response to the Planned Parenthood letter on Komen's behalf. It was steadfast, quietly resolute. Liz approved it—and insisted we loop in Hilary Rosen once again. Rosen continued to be Liz's touchstone when it came to gauging Planned Parenthood's reaction. Liz wanted to get Hilary's take on where things stood. By now I was beginning to have serious doubts about Rosen's analysis—that Planned Parenthood would observe our gentle-ladies' agreement not to take the issue to the media.

We let Hilary know that Liz wanted to speak with her. When the meeting request arrived, I was shocked to see that Emily Lenzner, whom we understood to work with Planned Parenthood, was included. Emily worked directly with Leslie, and despite Hilary earlier saying she was the Planned Parenthood expert and that she would connect us, that never occurred. I immediately let Liz know of my concerns. If indeed Emily worked with Planned Parenthood, it seemed highly inappropriate for her to be on a call during which we would be briefed on Planned Parenthood and its current thought process and discuss Komen's next steps. I recognized that Liz appreciated Hilary's counsel but I implored her to realize the risk.

Liz's response was short and alarming. She noted that she was deeply disappointed but not surprised and that she suspected that Emily may have been on most calls all along, even if she had not been announced.

Liz could have said a lot of things, but I doubt anything could have shocked me more. I did not know what to make of Liz's comments. What I did know was that I could not understand why no one else was troubled.

By now the leaks were running both ways. On January 8, 2012, the American Family Association radio show *Focal Point* reported that Komen was cutting grants to Planned Parenthood. I thought that this leak had come from within Komen. But who? I suppose it could have been someone sympathetic to the pro-life cause, but that didn't seem to make too much sense given the time that had passed. As I think back, I now wonder if someone who was familiar with our agreement not to go the press leaked the information purposely to the pro-life radio host in an effort to light the fuse and put Komen on the spot for breaking its word.

Regardless, I felt certain: war was only a matter of time. If the pro-life community had our granting information and declared it a "winnable issue"—as *Focal Point* had put it—Planned Parenthood would likely go nuclear. That's what I told Liz and Nancy. I thought that Hilary needed to reach out to Planned Parenthood. I thought that if she was who she said she was, had the contacts she claimed to have, and was really on Komen's side, she should have the ability to neutralize anything negative from this.

Liz had a conflict for the call, so I called Hilary directly. The very first issue I raised was my concern about SKDKnickerbocker representing both Komen and Planned Parenthood. Hilary responded that I did not need to worry. They kept a "firewall" between clients. *Firewall* was the exact word Hilary used. Next, I specifically asked where things stood with Planned Parenthood. She said that it was her sense that Planned Parenthood had decided not to fight the issue. They were standing down, she said. Again, "standing down" was the phrase she used. She said that we should let the story pass without any comment.

I relayed my conversation with Hilary to Liz, and all Liz said was that time would tell.

For the next two weeks, there was silence. Komen proceeded based on our understanding with Planned Parenthood—that we would still coordinate messaging and that neither organization would go to the press proactively. The two weeks of silence would prove to be the calm before the storm.

Because then, everything exploded.

6

Once a Bully,
Always a Bully

Komen had given millions of dollars in grants to Planned Par-enthood over the past two decades. The two organizations had always worked well together—our respective leadership sharing the same stages, attending the same events. Nancy Brinker had once held a position on a local Planned Parenthood board. There was a mutual respect and friendship—or so we thought. That's why we believed we would be able to work something out.

But, like the girlfriend of a guy with a history of broken relationships, we should have known better.

Planned Parenthood likes to call itself a women's health organization and, more recently, a cancer organization—shifting how it describes its mission to fit what the situation or political dynamic calls for. But Planned Parenthood is neither—at least according to its own stated mission. That mission—its "reason for being," says: "Planned Parenthood believes in the fundamental right of each individual, throughout the world, to manage his or her fertility, regardless of the individual's income, marital status, race, ethnicity, sexual orientation, age, national origin, or residence. . . . We believe that reproductive self-determination must be voluntary and preserve the individual's right to privacy. . . ."[1]

I think a strong case can be made that Planned Parenthood's "reason for being" goes far beyond contraception and abortion. It lives for liberal politics and lives by government funding. Since 1989, when its political arm was formed, Planned Parenthood has established itself as an integral part of the liberal policy machine and a deeply cynical exploiter of political conflict. In 2008, Planned Parenthood's CEO, Cecile Richards, made her political goals clear: "We aim to be the largest kick-butt political organization."[2]

Most people associate Planned Parenthood with its national network of abortion and birth control clinics. Today Planned Parenthood is a complex labyrinth of scores of affiliated lobbying organizations, political action committees (or PACs), and even 527s, Super PACs, and independent expenditure organizations. Together these organizations have spent millions in support of Democratic candidates, the Democratic Governors Association, the Democratic National Committee, and in working to put Democrats into the White House. Over the past ten years, Planned Parenthood has built an army of militant liberal ideologues ready to take up arms when called to action. With this kind of political clout and coin, Cecile has a seat at the table with President Obama, and Planned Parenthood is a trusted ally of the Democratic Party.

Planned Parenthood has more than a seat at the table. It is highly influential in determining who actually sits at the head of that table, actively engaging in numerous political campaigns—

almost exclusively for Democrats—for Congress and even the White House. In 2008, Planned Parenthood endorsed Barack Obama and actively campaigned for him.[3] Planned Parenthood endorsed Obama for a second a term as well, and is campaigning aggressively to ensure that he secures four more years in the White House.

Government Sustenance

Planned Parenthood is a major beneficiary of *our* tax dollars. According to its 2009–2010 Annual Report, Planned Parenthood's government haul is nearly $500 million a year in government payouts and reimbursements.[4] With government funding accounting for nearly 50 percent of its total annual revenues, Planned Parenthood achieves a certain degree of legitimacy it would not otherwise have. The significant percentage of government dollars also lends strong credence to the long-standing argument that federal dollars subsidize Planned Parenthood's abortion business. Today, Planned Parenthood is poised to secure even more government funding.

At the end of June, the Supreme Court of the United States (SCOTUS) upheld most elements of the Affordable Care Act, also known as Obamacare. With this ruling, Planned Parenthood has set its sights on several more government troughs from which to feed. Cecile Richards, local Planned Parenthood executives, and its supporters responded to the SCOTUS decision quickly and jubilantly, hailing it as a win for women—and Planned Parenthood.

Planned Parenthood aggressively promotes itself as a leading provider of primary health care for women. Yet, Planned Parenthood's annual report and fact sheets continue to emphasize that the "core" of its medical services are sexual and reproductive health care.[5] There is no mention of primary-care services. While a few local Planned Parenthood clinics, mostly in California, offer primary-care services, these services represent a tiny percentage of total services. Planned Parenthood no doubt is eager to replicate this model. Imagine the revenue opportunities for Planned Parenthood as a recognized primary-care provider. This would establish the nation's leading abortion provider as a primary gateway to the health-care system under Obamacare— thereby expanding its reach and revenue opportunities vastly.

Even without being recognized as a primary-care provider, Planned Parenthood stands to gain under Obamacare. Nearly all insurance plans must provide contraceptives without a co-pay. Contraception services account for about one-third of its total services (according to Planned Parenthood's most recent annual report). Clearly, Planned Parenthood benefits financially from this mandate—and one can see clearly why Cecile Richards aggressively lobbied for it. And, before anyone jumps to the conclusion that I am against all contraception, let me say that I am not. What I am against is forcing this mandate on religious organizations. It is a flagrant infringement on religious liberty and conscience. I also question why contraceptives would be available without co-pays when actual life-saving medicines, such as drugs to combat high blood pressure and diabetes or to treat cancer, are not.

Planned Parenthood has other significant revenue opportunities under Obamacare. The overhaul calls for extensive marketing, promotion, and outreach activities with tens of millions of dollars in grants to administer these programs in every state up for grabs. Planned Parenthood is already working to position itself as "uniquely qualified" to deliver these services.[6] Obamacare also establishes programs for enrollment assistance and patient navigators. Planned Parenthood is making a play to provide these services too—and secure even more of our tax dollars.

However, most disturbing, is the fact that Obamacare will provide coverage for abortions, despite the president's commitment that it would not. Under a rule issued by the U.S. Department of Health and Human Services, insurance plans within the state health exchanges are required to cover abortions. This means that Americans who oppose abortion and who are now required to have insurance (or pay a penalty) are put in the untenable position of having to choose between their beliefs and their health.

The new rule requires that an individual enrolled in one of these plans pay a separate fee of at least one dollar—an abortion surcharge. The abortion surcharge is paid directly to the abortion fund, going to an account that is separate from the monthly insurance premium. Why two separate accounts? It's the Obama administration's cunning and deceptive way to circumvent the prohibition of federal funds going to abortion—and no doubt, Planned Parenthood, given Cecile Richards' self-proclaimed deep involvement in shaping Obamacare, was in on this scheme too.

Pro-abortion proponents defend this abortion mandate, saying that no one is being *required* to choose a plan that covers elective abortions; they have the option to select another plan. Indeed, states must ensure that at least one plan in the exchange does not cover abortions. But there are a few catches.

First, insurers are prohibited from advertising about the surcharge. The liberal blog *Huffington Post* describes it as follows: "For people who opt into a health plan that covers abortion, the Affordable Care Act requires that health plans 'provide a notice to enrollees' at the time of enrollment that their plan includes the surcharge, but those plans are not allowed to advertise the specific surcharge." That's right—"not allowed." And, this from the administration that promised to be the most transparent in history.

Second, insurance companies are not permitted to disclose details about the one-dollar surcharge in literature about the plans. Instead, only the total cost of the premium can be advertised. The abortion surcharge is noted in the fine print of the plan document. But my question is this: if the insurer is prohibited from advertising about the surcharge, how would anyone know to look for it or ask about it?[7]

Government funding is life-sustaining nourishment for Planned Parenthood, and it wants more. Thanks to Obamacare, Planned Parenthood now has access to a never-ending feast. It's no wonder Cecile Richards took such an active role in shaping Obama's health-care reform package and why she is working so hard to ensure a second term for him. The debate over tax-dollar subsidies of Planned Parenthood's abortion operations no doubt will continue and likely intensify, given the opportunities for

Planned Parenthood to secure even more government funding. The abortion surcharge will also sharpen this debate.

But in addition to arguing that taxpayers should not be forced to subsidize an organization that provides abortions—an organization at the center of one of our country's most controversial issues—there is another case to be made. Our tax dollars bankroll Planned Parenthood's decidedly partisan, left-leaning political activities and agenda. This should disturb us all, particularly since we are asked to back their political play with our tax dollars.

None of this, though, was our concern at Komen. In fact, I had no idea how far Planned Parenthood's political tentacles reached, and I doubt anyone else at Komen knew, either. Our dealings with Planned Parenthood also had nothing whatsoever to do with abortion, although those of us at Komen National were surprised to learn that, in some of the community grants— and contrary to previous Komen statements—dollars were going to general administrative costs.

As we considered the next steps with Planned Parenthood, what we should have considered is this: Planned Parenthood had a huge stake in being recognized for something more than abortions. Planned Parenthood had a vested interest in ensuring that Democrats won—that the White House remained in the hands of Democrats. Millions of dollars in existing government funding and robust new streams of government dollars were at risk. Planned Parenthood's very survival depended on it, and there was no way that an organization as ruthless as Planned Parenthood with so much on the line was going to let Komen walk away free and clear. If Komen was successful, Planned Parenthood's opponents would be emboldened, and other entities that desired to be on neutral ground in the abortion debate would perhaps be inspired to make their own move.

Previous Attacks

Planned Parenthood has targeted other funding partners before. In 1990, AT&T decided it would no longer fund Planned Parenthood. The telecom giant wanted to get Planned Parenthood's politics off of its plate. "Much to our regret, Planned Parenthood has raised the level of political advocacy," then-chairman Robert Allen said to shareholders. "As a result, AT&T has become tainted and tarnished." For twenty-five years, AT&T gave Planned Parenthood $50,000 per year for teen educational town halls. Pro-life opponents sent letters and made calls to AT&T protesting the relationship.

Sure enough, Planned Parenthood did what they do best: they called their political allies. New York City comptroller Elizabeth Holtzman threatened to work with the New York City Employees' Retirement System to sell their three million shares of AT&T stock if the company didn't back down. Planned Parenthood also took out a full-page ad in the *Los Angeles Times* stating, "Caving in to extremists, AT&T hangs up on Planned Parenthood."[8]

The ad had a familiar ring. It continued, "AT&T caved in to anti-choice extremists just weeks before the annual meeting at which the question was to be openly discussed and voted on by shareholders. And decided to leave teens at risk. The free exchange of information is basic to AT&T's communications business. By catering to a closed-minded minority intolerant of differing ideas, AT&T is working against its own best interests. It only encourages those who use bullying tactics to stop women of all ages from getting the information they need to make their own personal, private decisions. . . . AT&T has sent a message that education and family planning—the only safe and sure ways to reduce abortion—are unworthy of support. That's precisely what the anti-choice extremists want. To see their threats succeed. To silence discussion. And take away *all* our choices, one by one."[9]

The ad cost $40,000. They took out three other ads, just like it, in papers around the country, spending well over three times the total AT&T grant amount—all in an attempt to bully AT&T into submission. Protesters descended on the stockholders' meeting.[10] State senators complained. "I think this is a terrible sort of thing for a corporation to do," wrote one Democratic lawmaker. Planned Parenthood ripped AT&T for "corporate cowardice."[11]

The then-head of Planned Parenthood, Faye Wattleton, snagged media appearances on NBC's *Today*, the *CBS Morning News*, the *CBS Evening News*, and a bevy of other major shows. Senator Barbara Boxer (D-CA) spoke up on their behalf.

Why did Planned Parenthood do it this way? As Wattleton said, "There was no other option to take—and let me explain to you why. We had been in conversation with AT&T for a number of months—as a matter of fact, more than a year, about the concerns they had about the opposition. . . . We said to them, 'you can't avoid this by defunding. This is an issue that *will* not go away—it will only give life and strength to people who think that they can push you around. . . .' "[12]

AT&T weathered the storm. They took some hits but refused to capitulate. They're still around.

I studied how AT&T handled their "breakup" with Planned Parenthood and made sure that Brinker and Liz also saw the case study. I wanted everyone to know what was ahead—"eyes wide open," I said repeatedly. I warned that, if we made the decision to walk away, we had to see it through—we could not blink.

I don't know what Nancy and Liz really expected to happen. I suspect that both believed it would be different for Komen. We weren't "corporate cowards," as Planned Parenthood called businesses that discontinued funding. We were Planned Parenthood's "sisters" in the nonprofit world; women were our shared constituency.

While AT&T stood strong against the Planned Parenthood assault, Wal-Mart caved almost immediately. In 1999, Planned Parenthood threatened a boycott if Wal-Mart stopped selling Preven, a morning-after pill. This wasn't even a direct threat to Planned Parenthood, but that didn't stop them from bringing their weight to bear.

Other organizations have also challenged Planned Parenthood—and been able to withstand the heat. In addition to AT&T, according to Life Decisions International (LDI), at least 280 organizations have pulled their funding from Planned Parenthood, most recently Bob Evans Restaurants.[13] Between 1992 and 2011, LDI reports that Planned Parenthood saw corporate sponsors withdraw some $40 million worth of funding. In the research we did, we found that those organizations that were most successful in the public eye were those that simply stated that Planned Parenthood sponsorships didn't meet their basic goals. They avoided politics and stuck to the general purpose of the programs they wanted to fund and how their association with Planned Parenthood was harming their brand.

Our standby media statement—the one finally agreed to after weeks of rewrites and edits—hit these points and was not focused on the investigations angle that Hilary had offered in early December. Regrettably, however, the moment that Komen cited investigations publicly, Planned Parenthood was able to seize on that one comment and use it to marshal its forces. Since the episode, several of my reporter friends have confirmed to me that once investigations became the central theme of the initial Associated Press article—at Komen's own doing—we put the issue on the field of politics. We gave Planned Parenthood home-field advantage.

Political Planned Parenthood

Planned Parenthood is about politics as much as it is about abortion and reproductive health. Specifically, Planned Parenthood's politics is about money—government funding, actually, because without the government funds, Planned Parenthood would be forced to pursue a different revenue model. The rhetoric on health, and especially women, is a smoke screen to hide its underlying political agenda—ensuring the continued flow of nearly $1.5 million a day in government funding and to elect pro-

Planned Parenthood policy makers who, in turn, work tirelessly to keep the cash flowing.

When Planned Parenthood isn't handing out condoms loaded with QR codes—bar codes that automatically tell the world where you just had sex (seriously, there's an entire website devoted to this with the crass slogan "Sex that safe, should be shared")[14]—they're giving out cheap abortions. Well, not giving them out—abortions are a profit center for Planned Parenthood. In 2009, Live Action estimated that $155.5 million of Planned Parenthood's $404.9 million health center income (nongovernment funding) came from performing abortions—that's 38.4 percent of health-related, nongovernment revenue.[15]

That's a lot of money from abortion, but Planned Parenthood rakes in a lot of government money, too. Government subsidies represent just over 46 percent of Planned Parenthood's total annual revenues. Donations and non-abortion-related revenue account for only about 15 percent of its annual revenues.

Planned Parenthood is a 501(c)3 organization—a charitable nonprofit. It also spends in excess of $56 million on public policy.[16] Now, as a public policy person, I can tell you that not every dollar spent on public policy is spent on lobbying. But a significant percentage is. And the money spent on public policy and lobbying is just part of Planned Parenthood's overall political spending.

Planned Parenthood is a vast network of more than one hundred affiliated organizations at the local, state, and national level. Many of these entities are political in nature with various types of IRS tax status. The clinics themselves are generally nonprofit organizations. At the national level, Planned Parenthood Federation of America is the overarching charitable organization—the mother ship, if you will. Then there is the Planned Parenthood Action Fund, organized as a 501(c)4 entity, or a so-called grassroots advocacy organization. Cecile Richards is head of both organizations. Scores of Planned Parenthood PACs, 527 groups, and independent expenditure organizations combine to give Planned Parenthood serious political muscle—to actively engage in political campaigns, make financial contributions to candidates and political parties, endorse candidates, and even hit the campaign trail in support of specific (Democratic, of course) candidates.

While all of this may well follow the letter of the law, it is alarming that any organization funded to such a significant extent with *our* tax dollars can be so emphatically partisan and so deeply entrenched in political campaigning. Could you imagine the screams of protest if, say, the National Rifle Association were subsidized by the government to the extent of Planned Parenthood?

Planned Parenthood's viewpoint is unwaveringly and unapologetically leftist. Take, for example, the Pennsylvania primaries. Planned Parenthood engaged in a big way—through its Action Fund. The pink-plastered Women Are Watching website announced joyously in April 2012, "On Tuesday, advocates for women's health scored crucial victories in Pennsylvania primaries, overwhelmingly rejecting the attacks on women's health by far-right lawmakers this session. . . . This week's victories send an important message that politicians should keep politics out of the deeply personal decisions a woman makes in consultation with her family, her faith, and her doctor."[17]

The website has various sections, including "who we are watching" and "why we are watching." Planned Parenthood's "chumps" and "champs" feature is particularly revealing. The chumps, naturally, are all Republicans, while the champs are all Democrats. Planned Parenthood even prominently features the various candidates it has formally endorsed. A pink swag— Planned Parenthood's seal of approval—appears on the photos of Barack Obama, Jon Tester, Claire McCaskill, and others. Now, to be fair, Planned Parenthood has supported a few Republicans over the years, those who have been willing to support the organization's abortion-providing, tax-dollar-guzzling agenda, no questions asked. But take even one step out of line and Planned Parenthood turns on you. Just ask Congresswoman Susan Collins of Maine.

Through Planned Parenthood Votes, another one of its many political entities, the women's health charity poser spent $100,000 in TV ads in support of the Democrat for a seat in the Pennsylvania House of Representatives.[18] Planned Parenthood Wisconsin's political arm also engaged in the recall effort of Republican governor Scott Walker.

———

The bonds between Planned Parenthood and the Obama administration run deep. Cecile Richards isn't just the president of Planned Parenthood. She is President Obama's closest outside advisor on women's issues. She's also an open supporter—and surrogate—of President Obama in his reelection effort. On May 17, 2012, she cut a video for President Obama's reelection campaign; the campaign posted it with the headline "Why Cecile Richards has President Obama's back." Cecile looks into the camera and says, "As president of Planned Parenthood, I think about women's health care every day, and the health care for 3 million who turn to us each year. It's so important that women take a moment and pay attention to what's happening in this election, because the results are going to impact not only their lives, but the lives of their children for generations to come. In this election, there's a strong contrast between the positions of this president, who believes in women, who trusts women to make responsible decisions, and frankly the Republican Party leadership who seems to want to take away the right and put government in between women and their doctors.

"I think the thing that disturbed me, and really, frankly, hundreds of thousands of women who've contacted us since Mitt Romney said he was going to get rid of Planned Parenthood, is that he's putting politics ahead of women's health care access. Most of the women who come to Planned Parenthood come because they need preventive care access. They need access to affordable birth control, lifesaving cancer screenings and the kind of care we provide. For women, their health care doesn't come with a political label. The fact that we're actually having a fight in this country about whether women should have access to birth control is extraordinary. So it's been wonderful to have President Obama as a champion for access to health care for all women in this country.

"We've worked very hard with this administration to ensure that all women, regardless of their employer, could get access to birth control with no expensive copay or deductible. It's basic health care for women. Women are going to determine who the next president is. They take these decisions very seriously, and they have so much at stake in this election. And I think when women look at the positions of Mr. Romney, who really wants to take women back to the 1950s, and the record of President Obama and all that he has done for women and American families, there's a clear choice."[19]

Her video is full of misleading statements and even outright lies. First, Romney never said that he would "get rid of Planned Parenthood." He said he wanted to end federal funding for it. There's a big difference. Second, regarding Cecile's point about Romney wanting to take women back to the 1950s, this too is untrue and farfetched—there's no evidence to that proposition whatsoever. But then, Cecile is a master of hyperbole and distortion.

This summer, just before Romney secured the Republican nomination for president, Planned Parenthood launched a $1.4 million attack ad campaign against Romney. A Planned Parenthood spokesperson said the ads were just a "small down payment" on what was to come.[20] True to their word, Planned Parenthood has been aggressively campaigning on behalf of President Obama, slamming presumptive GOP nominee Mitt Romney at every turn. Cecile herself is the chief Obama cheerleader—an actual political surrogate for the campaign, traveling the country to rally her troops for her guy and to secure the continued flow of hundreds of millions of dollars in government funds to her organization.[21]

But the bigger point was exactly what Cecile said it was: Planned Parenthood regularly works with the Obama administration to achieve its goals. According to Jake Tapper of ABC News, Cecile Richards was one of President Obama's top advisors on forcing Catholic employers to provide health-care coverage including contraception. Melody Barnes, the former Domestic Policy Council director for the White House, was also part of the working group—and she had been a former Planned Parenthood Action Fund board member. When Obama finally made his decision about the Catholic contraception mandate, Obama called three people: Sister Carol Keehan of the Catholic Health Association, Cardinal-designate Timothy Dolan of New York, and Cecile Richards.[22]

Throughout Planned Parenthood's assault on Komen, my personal politics—and even Nancy's—were the focus of much airtime, ink, and ire. Cecile was given a full pass. Planned Parenthood's deep political connections and aggressive political campaigns were ignored. Cecile openly endorsed President Obama—and has been on the campaign trail for President Obama and various Democratic candidates. She spoke at the 2008 Democratic National Convention. Planned Parenthood is even prominently featured in Obama campaign ads. None of this was mentioned by mainstream media. There was never even a mention of the fact that Cecile is the daughter of the late Ann Richards, who was a Democratic governor of Texas.

I've learned a lot about Planned Parenthood since that last Monday in January when the abortion provider opened fire on

Komen. I knew about the arguments that every dollar of government funding freed up a dollar for abortion services. But I think that the government subsidies do even more than that. The government subsidies that Planned Parenthood receives enable it to free up dollars that are then shifted from its nonprofit work to its political work. With considerable government dollars flowing in, Planned Parenthood can focus much of its fund-raising efforts on its political mission. Each year, Planned Parenthood's 501(c)3 "donates" millions of dollars from its budget to its 501(c)4—as a gift. Planned Parenthood's 2010 form 990, filed with the IRS, shows that Planned Parenthood granted $6.5 million to its Action Fund. They gave that entity almost $100,000 just for shared facilities. Another $3.1 million was used to cover Action Fund employees' salaries, and another $3.3 million to reimburse another organization's services. Essentially this is a legalized scheme in which Planned Parenthood takes in nearly $500 million a year in government money and hundreds of millions more in other revenue—contributions and payments for services—and then turns a significant portion of these funds over to its political arm to support Democrats in order to keep the money well pumping.

Komen also has a 501(c)4 for lobbying and grassroots advocacy purposes—the Komen Advocacy Alliance—and we also sent money from the 501(c)3 to the 501(c)4; about $2.5 million per year. But there are significant differences. First, Komen does not receive nearly 50 percent of its annual revenues from government funding—Komen is not subsidized by government funding. Second, Komen is strictly nonpartisan in its activities—never favoring one party or candidate over another. Komen focuses specifically on issues related to the fight against breast cancer. There is no political campaigning by Komen as an organization—not through its advocacy entity, by Nancy Brinker, or by anyone as a Komen employee. In fact, Nancy and I and others in senior management even stayed out of political activities personally as well—simply to avoid any questions or even the appearance of partisanship.

Planned Parenthood, through its Action Fund and scores of local political entities, makes it crystal clear where the organization's political heart lies. They spent millions during the last weeks of the 2000 election pushing ads against George W. Bush. During the 2004 election cycle, Planned Parenthood spent about $1.6 million via its PAC; it spent millions more on "public policy" that amounted to little more than advertising for the Democratic Party. Democrats received 95 percent of its PAC spending. In 2008, Planned Parenthood took in $454,642; 99 percent went to Democrats. Together these organizations spent millions in the 2008 and 2010 election cycles—including almost $1 million in independent expenditures in 2010. The beneficiaries of these dollars were, of course, almost all Democrats.[23]

Planned Parenthood is gearing up for the 2012 elections, too. As of the spring of 2012, the Planned Parenthood Action Fund PAC had raised nearly $500,000, while the 527 entity, Planned Parenthood Votes, had amassed a war chest of nearly $1.2 million.[24]

The Planned Parenthood Action Fund has almost nothing to do with the broader issues of women's health. Although the websites are awash in breast cancer pink, you'll be hard-pressed to find much information on breast cancer. Instead the focus is on abortion and contraception, almost to the exclusion of all else.

SKDKnickerbocker also has deep ties to the Democratic Party and, in particular, to President Obama. An entire page on the liberal PR firm's website is devoted to bragging about its "far-reaching role" in electing Obama.[25] Planned Parenthood, Rosen's firm SKDKnickerbocker, and the Obama administration share a lot more than ideology. Key staffers have worked for one or the other at some point. It's a virtual revolving door when it comes to personnel. In November 2011, a top White House aide was named to a senior position at Planned Parenthood.[26] Just recently, Planned Parenthood's media outreach person was named a deputy secretary at the U.S. Department of Health and Human Services. Anita Dunn, a key principal alongside Rosen at SKDKnickerbocker, is Obama's former communications director.

Cecile herself worked for Nancy Pelosi for years—coincidentally alongside Komen PR consultant Brendan Daly. Even when Pelosi and other political players engaged against Komen, no one in the media raised Cecile's politics or her political connections as issues. Yet Sarah Palin's endorsement of my gubernatorial run was played up over and over again as part of the news coverage of Planned Parenthood's mugging of Komen, used as "evidence" that my politics was central to the decision.

Do Cecile's activities across the charitable entity and the various political organizations cross any lines? Is Planned Parenthood breaking any laws? Who knows. But with so many organizations and such blatant and aggressive partisan political activities—and even a cadre of "political and organizing directors,"[27] it would seem to be worth examining—especially when so much of our tax dollars are involved.

What is clear is to me is that Planned Parenthood is far more about politics than it is about breast cancer or even women's health, for that matter. The noncontroversial themes are pushed to take the focus off abortion, and these softer themes serve as a veil to hide the truth: Planned Parenthood is the front man—or woman, if you will—for the Democratic Party and the liberal agenda.

The "War on Women"

Planned Parenthood had been under scrutiny from conservatives who do not support Americans' funding the country's leading abortion provider for some time. However, with the 2010 elections, that scrutiny intensified. Democrats managed to cling to a majority in the U.S. Senate. President Obama lost his Democratic majority in the House of Representatives, and his poor economic record had not won Americans to his side. In fact, his economic record was abysmal, especially for women. The president promised hope, but many, particularly women, simply found despair. Nine out of every ten people who lost jobs under Obama between January 2009 and March 2012 were female.[28]

In 2008, Obama won the male vote over his Republican opponent, Senator John McCain (R-AZ), by a slim margin of 49 percent to 48 percent—but he cleaned up among women, winning 56 percent to 43 percent. In 2010, for the first time in years, Republicans won a majority of the female vote. By the end of 2011, Obama's approval ratings had slipped dramatically among men—so much so that a poll pitting him against presumptive Republican presidential nominee Mitt Romney put him a shocking 20 percentage points down among men. Obama still maintained a 6-point lead among women, but this was far from the 13-point lead he had in 2008.[29]

Clearly, Obama had to boost his position with women to have a chance of maintaining the presidency. So Democratic political strategists, such as Hilary Rosen and others, latched on to the so-called war on women as a political campaign theme and tagged Republicans as the aggressors.

But Obama needed more than that. The debate had to be about more than just abortion. The "war on women" had to be broader—focused on something that would energize women beyond the traditional pro-abortion wedge issue that has long divided women and America in general. And, of course, with the nation's continued high unemployment rates, Obama wanted to talk about anything but the economy. If Republican leaders, most of whom are men, could be painted as sexists and out of touch with today's women, there might be an opening. And, brilliantly, contraceptives were added to the mix.

President Obama had Planned Parenthood as a powerful ally. They sounded the clarion call and readied their devout followers for war. The timing of Komen's decision to part ways with Planned Parenthood was fortuitous. It enabled Planned Parenthood to plan the timing of its attack to most benefit Obama and

Democrats in this crucial election year, adding another layer to the "war on women" argument. And the Democrats were aided by several unforced errors on the part of Republicans. Komen's timing could not have been worse for us and better for Obama, the Democrats, and Planned Parenthood. I believe that Komen became an unwitting and convenient pawn used to elevate the "war on women." There were just too many coincidences.

The Obama administration clashes with the Catholic Church over mandated insurance coverage for contraception. Republican presidential candidate Rick Santorum, who had made social issues the hallmark of his campaign, began to gain traction right about that time. Women's health was headline news. Komen's commonsense decision was suddenly caught up in a debate on conscience and contraception and what the Democrats said was a war on women.

Hilary Rosen, our chosen consultant, was visiting the White House on a regular basis. Thanks to leaks from inside Komen, Cecile became aware of our decision in early December, about two weeks before Liz informed her directly in mid-December. It is well documented that Hilary and Cecile maintain a close relationship with the White House. Both visited the White House numerous times in December leading up to the January 30 launch of Planned Parenthood's war on Komen. I wonder just what was discussed between Obama administration officials, SKDKnickerbocker, and its client, the Democratic National Committee.

In the January 6, 2012, Republican primary debate, ABC's George Stephanopoulos, former Clinton administration top staffer and noted hit man for the Democratic left in the press, asked a bizarre question. "Governor Romney," he blurted, "do you believe that states have the right to ban contraception? Or is that trumped by a constitutional right to privacy?"

The question itself was strange, out of left field. Since the 1960s, it has been illegal under relevant U.S. Supreme Court rulings for a state to ban contraception. Romney himself was taken aback by the question. "George," he said, "this is an unusual topic that you're raising. . . . Given that there's no state that wants to do so, and I don't know of any candidate that wants to do so, you're asking could it constitutionally be done?"

But Stephanopoulos didn't want an answer. He wanted to make a point. "Do you believe states have that right or not?" he reiterated.

"George," Romney answered, "I don't know if the state has a right to ban contraception, no state wants to! The idea of you putting forward things that states *might* want to do, that no state wants to do, and then asking me whether they can do it or not is kind of a silly thing."

It was more than silly—because just two weeks later, the other shoe dropped. On January 20, with the backing of Planned Parenthood and assistance from Cecile Richards as one of the president's women's health advisors, the Obama administration announced that religious employers would have to provide health coverage including contraceptives. Quickly termed the contraceptive mandate, the issue blew up in the public sphere, with most Americans opposing the mandate on religious liberty grounds.

But there was a larger point that the Obama campaign seemed to be pursuing. They had to pick a fight over contraception. They wanted to paint conservatives as regressive Neanderthals trying to stop women from having access to contraception. If that meant picking a fight with the Catholic Church, so be it. Planned Parenthood was more than happy to join the fight. If the mandate became law, it opened up a steady new revenue stream for them.

Komen versus Planned Parenthood would be a perfect conflict, setting up an epic girl fight, featuring what the press called conservative crazies (that would be Nancy and me) and advancing the war on women. Komen would be portrayed as a right-wing organization out to victimize women on behalf of a radical religious, pro-life agenda.

Planned Parenthood had its plan, and I believe it had been in the works since the very first leak from Komen to Planned Parenthood. Here's what else I believe: Cecile never intended to proceed amicably. Planned Parenthood had what it needed for an effective offensive: an inside source at Komen, a Komen senior executive with a public pro-life record, a Komen CEO who was a well-known Republican, and Komen's misplaced sense of loyalty to a longtime grantee and mistaken belief that a peaceful transition was possible.

Then, like dominoes falling, events toppled on one another. The contraception mandate announcement was made on January 20. On January 22, the thirty-ninth anniversary of *Roe v.*

Wade, President Obama himself announced that "we must . . . continue our efforts to ensure that our daughters have the same rights, freedoms, and opportunities as our sons to fulfill their dreams." Cecile stated, "In the general election, there will be a stark contrast between the GOP nominee and the president on a fundamental issue important to women: birth control. Women's health is a key issue for women voters, who will likely decide the next election. And the more the GOP presidential candidates attack women's health, the more out of sync they are with women voters."[30] Cecile knew she couldn't make the "war on women" only about abortion—it had to be about contraception, access to which was widely supported. By focusing on women's health more broadly, perhaps women and the American public generally could be led into believing that there really was an assault on women. In doing so, the pro-life battle against abortion and a separate battle for religious freedom would be overshadowed.

What Planned Parenthood—along with the Democratic Party, the White House, the media—was about to unleash on Komen was a true war on women. For their own political and money motives, they were willing to demonize Komen, along with Nancy and me personally. It would be portrayed as a women's health organization (Komen) cravenly bowing to right-wing power (me) in order to harm low-income women.

The plan was executed flawlessly, with vicious effectiveness. The actors played their parts to perfection. It was as brilliant as it was despicable. To me there were just too many coincidences for it all to have been simple happenstance.

Just days after Obama made his contraception announcement, two days after Cecile and the administration celebrated the thirty-ninth anniversary of *Roe v. Wade*, Komen received a call from the head of the Democratic National Committee. That call kicked off one of the most contemptible acts of coordinated bullying in modern American political history.

7

Taken Hostage

On January 24, 2012, just a few weeks after we had received what I thought was our warning shot from Cecile Richards, Planned Parenthood bought a building in New York City for its headquarters. The cost: $34.8 million. Planned Parenthood had already been renting the space, which spanned a whopping 104,000 square feet. Now it owned this expensive Manhattan real estate.[1] New York City, at the same time, even pledged $15 million in bond funding for renovations to the building.[2] New York City mayor Michael Bloomberg would later personally pledge $250,000 to Planned Parenthood to help make up the supposed deficit created by the loss of the Komen grants. As of June 30, 2010, according to its most recent annual report, Planned Parenthood showed total net assets of more than $1.2 billion.[3]

Clearly, Planned Parenthood could get along without Komen and its $680,000 in annual grants—grants that represented far less than one percent of its total budget. Komen's grant dollars were inconsequential to Planned Parenthood's financial status and its mission. Their cries of poverty—their dire claims about not being able to care for low-income women because of losing less than $700,000 a year in potential future grants—seemed disingenuous and grossly overstated next to a real estate expenditure roughly fifty times as large, and annual revenues in excess of $1 billion per year.

But I never thought Planned Parenthood was about breast cancer services or helping low-income women.

It was about politics, pure and simple.

The Democratic Party Connection

It was now January 23. It had been more than two weeks since we'd heard anything at all from Planned Parenthood or, as far as I knew, from Hilary Rosen. The issue, it seemed, was dormant.

That day, however, I received a message from the office of Representative Debbie Wasserman Schultz (D-FL), chairwoman of the Democratic National Committee. The message said that Representative Wasserman Schultz had to speak to Nancy Brinker "urgently"—that day if possible. We followed up, but for two days there was no response. I called and emailed repeatedly. Finally, her office responded that the congresswoman wanted to speak to Nancy about a personal matter and that the call had been scheduled with Nancy's office directly.

As it turned out, the call was now scheduled for January 30. That "urgent" request to speak immediately could now wait for an entire week. That seemed strange, suspicious. The timing of this call would be yet another coincidence.

I had the feeling that the call was about Planned Parenthood, but Nancy disagreed initially. She seemed to take Wasserman Schultz at her word that it was indeed something personal. Still, I thought that Nancy needed to be prepared just in case the call was about Planned Parenthood. The more Nancy thought about it, the more she seemed to consider that the call was, indeed, about Planned Parenthood. She even wondered if it meant that Planned Parenthood was about to attack. But she seemed resolute in her decision, saying that Komen had every right to make grants for the highest and best purpose and expressing her dislike for pressure tactics. When Nancy told me that, if Wasserman Schultz pushed back, she would push right back in the nicest of ways, I thought that Nancy sounded like she was more than ready for the fight.

Nancy wanted to know if we had heard anything from Planned Parenthood. I hadn't heard a thing.

Nancy contacted Komen board member John Raffaelli, who had called his contact at Planned Parenthood back in December and received an encouraging report that Planned Parenthood would work with Komen. He seemed to have a good relationship with Planned Parenthood, and I'm guessing Nancy wanted some additional advice and to see if he had heard anything new. Nancy shared John's suggestions with me. He suggested that she try to soften the Planned Parenthood issue by explaining that we were redirecting money from education to treatment and testing; that many of our pro–Planned Parenthood board members were in favor of cutting the grants; that Komen had weathered storms on behalf of Planned Parenthood before, so this wasn't political. Nancy, it seemed, was preparing for an emotional hailstorm from Wasserman Schultz and said that she hoped the congress-woman's tone wasn't too strong, noting that they had been good donors and friends. I wasn't sure if Nancy meant she had been a good donor and friend to Wasserman Schultz or that Komen had been a good donor and friend to Planned Parenthood—perhaps it was both, I thought.

The battle lines were softly being drawn. Ironically, Liz had been in Ohio for a series of meetings, including one with the bishop of Cleveland. She discussed Komen's new grant policies with him and the effect on Planned Parenthood. I know because she asked me to prepare a briefing paper for the bishop, so that he could take it with him to Rome for upcoming meetings at the Vatican. When Liz followed up with me about her meeting, she remarked that the bishop was a really nice man. I thought she sounded surprised.

The Media Connection

On January 30, Hilary Rosen was in the Komen D.C. office, meeting with Leslie Aun. I would learn about this meeting from Liz late that afternoon. I had no idea about Leslie's meeting with Hilary and others from SKDKnickerbocker. I remember thinking it very peculiar that Rosen was physically in our office and that Leslie had failed to mentioned it. I would have thought a short status meeting regarding Planned Parenthood would have been scheduled, or at the very least, that Leslie would have ensured a personal introduction—since I had yet to actually meet Hilary in person. But I had not heard from Hilary in weeks, and I don't think Liz had, either, because it was her practice to update me.

Sometime late that morning, another curious thing happened. Actually, it was more than just curious—it was a bombshell. Leslie texted me that she had been contacted by an Associated Press reporter who said he was doing a story on Komen and Planned Parenthood. We would soon learn that he knew everything about the situation—from Planned Parenthood's point of view. He indicated that he had talked with Cecile and even knew the details of Liz's private call with Cecile.

There were other peculiarities from that day. How ironic that Associated Press called on the very same day that the head of the Democratic National Committee had scheduled a call with Nancy. How ironic that Associated Press called while Hilary Rosen and others from SKDKnickerbocker, including the firm's Planned Parenthood expert, were actually in the Komen office. More coincidences.

Our strategy—developed with Ogilvy, Rosen, the Komen communications team, and the management team—was to issue a magnanimous statement and weather the storm. The less we said, we figured, the lower the risk of being pulled into a detailed debate about the merits of Planned Parenthood.

I let Liz know that afternoon about the call from Associated Press and provided her with a copy of the press statement with a few additional changes, given the apparent direction Planned Parenthood was now taking. The statement focused on our granting strategies, that women were our highest priority, and that it was regrettable when changes in strategic priorities affected any of our grantees, particularly a long-standing partner like Planned Parenthood. While others had reviewed the statement one last time, I wanted Liz to have a final look, as well. She said that the statement was very strong.

I responded that I was putting the final statement in Leslie's hands and reminding her yet again that we were issuing a statement only.

I also suggested to Liz that a call to Hilary was in order. I thought that we should let Hilary know how disappointed we were to learn that Planned Parenthood had proactively gone to the press without so much as a heads-up that she had changed her mind. Liz's response caught me off guard. She said that she thought Hilary was in our D.C. office at that very moment—and she was right.

I headed down to the main conference room and, sure enough, there was Hilary, along with Leslie, and others from SKDKnickerbocker. I remain puzzled even today why Leslie had not mentioned that Hilary was in our office when she advised me of the Associated Press inquiry.

I asked Hilary if we could speak, and we proceeded to an office down the hall. I began to bring Hilary up to speed, but she quickly stopped me, saying that Leslie had already done so. I then asked for her assessment of the situation, asking if she thought Planned Parenthood was going to DEFCON 4. Seated in a chair across from me, Hilary looked me straight in the eye and with a smile said, "Oh no, I don't think this is any big deal." I was taken aback by her response, because it sure felt like a big deal to me, but then Hilary was our expert on this. She went on to say something about Wall Street and the stock market being turned pink and that, since Cecile is a highly emotional person, this probably affected her. She added, "Sometimes, Cecile just goes rogue."

This would turn out to be so far off the mark as to raise serious questions for me. I did not really believe that the call was no big deal, but Hilary was our connection to Planned Parenthood; she had positioned herself as having direct contact with Cecile and other key executives. I know now that I should have acted—because the Associated Press reporter's call signaled the first offensive in Planned Parenthood's assault. Later that night, I realized my stupidity. I don't know if Nancy or Liz ever asked Hilary about her counsel and assessment of Planned Parenthood and its intentions. I can say that I sure would like to know how the advice from someone who was hired to manage issues on the left for Komen, someone whose firm included a Planned Parenthood expert (as Hilary had described Emily Lenzner) and billed itself as tightly wired with Planned Parenthood and its top executives, could be so completely off base.

We discussed our response, and Leslie and Rosen continued to push for full interviews, saying that reporters would be mad if they only received a statement. I think now that most at Komen would have preferred angry reporters over the firestorm that would be lit by this initial news story.

Late that same afternoon, Nancy spoke with Debbie Wasserman Schultz, the congresswoman from Florida and head of the Democratic National Committee.

I was now even more suspicious about the timing of this call.

Could this really be mere coincidence? Wasserman Schultz's office first called the previous Monday, saying it was imperative that she speak with Nancy that day. We tried to reach someone in the congressional office. When Wasserman Schultz's office finally returned our messages and scheduled the conversation, the call was delayed for nearly a week—to the same day that Associated Press called. Was it just happenstance the Wasserman Schultz's office had set the call for the very afternoon of the day of the Associated Press reporter's call?

Nothing was public about Komen's decision. The Associated Press story would not be out until the next day. Yet Wasserman Schultz knew about everything in great detail. Somehow she was privy to what had been going on within our organization. Nancy updated me on her call with Wasserman Schultz: Wasserman Schultz was particularly focused on the "investigations" angle. Nancy told her that our grant policy was a guideline that we followed, but Wasserman Schultz pushed back, saying that Planned Parenthood was always under investigation. Nancy tried to explain that Komen could not differentiate between investigations, but that our bigger concern was the sanctity of our grants and the need to have measurable outcomes—the kind of meaningful outcomes that the Planned Parenthood grants simply did not provide. Nancy said she told Wasserman Schultz that Komen would not be bullied because we needed to evolve our grants.

When Nancy recounted the call, she said it was a long one and that it was extremely ugly in its tone. Wasserman Schultz, she said, had told her that Komen would regret the decision. According to Nancy, Wasserman Schultz raised one additional issue: me. I wrote down precisely what Nancy said Wasserman Schultz had said: "How dare you hire someone who was diametrically opposed to Planned Parenthood."

There had now been two disquieting coincidences that day—and as I've said, I don't really believe in coincidences. First, Hilary just happened to be in the office the day Planned Parenthood went to Associated Press, and the day Associated Press called us. Second, Wasserman Schultz just happened to have a prescheduled call set with Nancy on the same day as well.

Members of Congress often make calls in support of their constituents. What bothered me—and should bother anyone—about the Wasserman Schulz call was the timing and the tone that Nancy described. Nancy can hold her own, but it was clear by her description that Wasserman Schultz had been overbearing, if not threatening. Was it appropriate for a sitting member of Congress and the head of the DNC to browbeat a private organization about its grants and who would get them? The timing of the call seemed to suggest that if Komen would just continue the Planned Parenthood grants, all would be forgiven—that if Komen got back in line, the bullies would back off.

Prelude to Destruction

The ground war had been declared. The leftist army was preparing to strike.

As I said, Komen's plan was to simply issue the written statement—no proactive media outreach and no interviews. Nevertheless, Leslie and Rosen continued to press the idea that Leslie "had" to do on-the-record interviews. Ari Fleischer's efforts to recruit a senior communications person had faltered. I thought it was a bad idea for Leslie to be on the phone with the reporter—any reporter—let alone one who was going to be antagonistic; one who had been prepared diligently by Cecile to ask the most aggressive questions.

Leslie actually came to me that day, before she had responded in any way to Associated Press—at least she said she had not responded yet. She seemed a bit nervous. She never mentioned that Hilary was in our offices, though she of course knew that Hilary was our point person with Planned Parenthood. "First," I reminded her, "you're not to do an interview. We have all agreed that it's a statement only." At this point she only had an email from the reporter—she said he'd provided no details. So, I suggested, "Just find out what he knows, but *remember,* no interview. Feel him out. Then we will have the benefit of a better understanding of the direction he's taking and can convene the team if needed." The idea was obvious: Do what communications people do. First, get the scope and direction of the story and pull background on the reporter. Get your team together to review the plan and response. Adjust if necessary. It was Media Relations 101 not to do an interview cold if it could be avoided.

And yet for reasons I will never comprehend, in between her meetings with Rosen and after our specific conversation in which I reiterated Liz's directions, Leslie did a stone-cold interview with the Associated Press reporter.

In the interview, rather than sticking to our standby statement, Leslie referred to the document we had used to guide our local affiliates on how to administer grants—a document that was *never* intended for use with the media. The papers themselves referenced that they were not for external distribution. We had agreed: a short, straightforward statement that would allow us to take the high road and that focused on our mission.

I don't know why Leslie did the interview, given that Komen's agreed-upon response had been to issue the statement. I also don't know why she used the affiliate granting guidelines Q&A for a press interview or why she didn't get more information and confer with her colleagues. When she came down to my office and told me she had done the interview, I was shocked. When I asked why, she just said, "Oh, my bad."

That evening, Leslie emailed the entire team about her interview with Associated Press. She noted that the reporter wrote frequently about women and social issues; about abortion.

After she'd done the interview, Leslie pulled background on the reporter. He was a Planned Parenthood ally. A February 2011 article he'd written about Planned Parenthood was an approving portrayal of the organization, quoting Cecile at length. "Planned Parenthood leaders and allies are seizing the moment to rally support," David Crary gushed, "saying the ultimate target of the attacks [from the pro-life community] is the ability of American women to get the reproductive health services they desire. . . . Through its affiliates, Planned Parenthood operates more than 800 clinics and health centers across the U.S., serving more than 3 million patients a year." The article was essentially a rehashed Planned Parenthood press release.[4]

In her recap, Leslie said that it was her assessment that the reporter had talked directly to Cecile Richards and was sympathetic to her and Planned Parenthood. She specifically noted that she had never spoken to a national reporter who was so openly biased. His first words, according to Leslie, were that he was writing a story about Komen cutting off funding to Planned Parenthood and wanted to know if Komen was giving in to pressure from right-to-lifers.

Undaunted by the fact that this was a deeply biased reporter who seemed ready to shred Komen, Leslie forged on. Why she didn't stop, find a way to get off the call, so that we could pull the team together to reassess, I do not know. The focus of the interview was the investigations—precisely the point that Wasserman Schultz and Cecile had focused on in their attempt to turn Komen's basic business decision into a political one.

Leslie continued to provide a blow-by-blow of the interview. She said he wanted additional details about the congressional investigation and that she did her best to downplay the situation. Yet she sent him a copy of the September 15 House Energy and Commerce Committee letter to Planned Parenthood. I could not understand how feeding the reporter information about the congressional investigation helped Komen or downplayed the situation. In providing the letter, it seemed to me that we were inadvertently escalating the investigations issue. I also did not understand why Leslie followed the reporter down the investigations path. Even if the reporter was asking questions on the investigations angle, why wasn't she pivoting to *our* messages? Komen was evolving its granting strategy in order to do more and do better by women, and unfortunately, our new strategy did affect Planned Parenthood. Period.

Leslie's update wrapped up as follows: She wasn't certain when the story would appear but predicted that it would be heavily slanted in Planned Parenthood's favor. She added that she thought this was unfortunate because she couldn't see how this publicity served Planned Parenthood's interest. She also said that she had been getting intel that Planned Parenthood did not intend to go public and that it might be a case of Cecile having gone rogue. She concluded with her assessment that no experienced communications person would condone this strategy.

Interestingly, Leslie's report parroted Rosen's assessment of the current situation to me from earlier that afternoon—nearly word for word.

As I said, I really don't know why Leslie did the interview or why it was handled the way it was. It didn't really matter at this point. The result was the same: Komen was now directly in the line of fire. Planned Parenthood had exactly what it needed to set us up as political culprits, and Komen would become a casualty in the world of cutthroat election-year campaigning, as Democrats sought to push the politically motivated war on women.

Even today, I still have a sinking feeling about Leslie, someone I had come to consider a friend. Why did she do that interview? She was an experienced communications person, so I couldn't understand how the interview turned out the way it did. With Hilary in the office, did she and Leslie decide to go with a different strategy? Leslie would send me a text message after my resignation, repeating something I had once said to her when she asked me about how I dealt with the cruelties of the media during my campaign. Her message said, "A wise woman once told me that no one gets to define you. You define yourself."

That was it. I wonder to this day why she sent that and what it meant.

Once the investigations issue became the central theme of our message, there was no taking it back. We were already off the rails—something several reporters I know would later confirm. Everyone waited with apprehension for the Associated Press story.

The tsunami was coming—we all knew it, but like people trapped on the island in its path, there was little we could do. The direction the story would take was set. The first large waves hit shore that evening. Calls from Planned Parenthood supporters were starting—and the Associated Press story was not even out yet. Katrina McGhee, Komen's marketing head, pointed out that the Facebook pages of our corporate partners would likely be next.

I agreed with that, and based on the note, thought Katrina and her team would begin monitoring our sponsors' Facebook pages. I also thought the communications team would be trolling the Internet, watching for any sign that might give us early warning. It would turn out that this was not happening. This was what I meant when I said earlier that I had been made the "conductor" of an orchestra that didn't play.

I later found out that on Monday—*prior* to the Associated Press story breaking—a pro–Planned Parenthood blog called *Shakespeare's Sister* posted that Komen was dropping its Planned Parenthood grants. The post blended fact with fiction and also contained confidential information that could only have come from within Komen offices . . . or from Planned Parenthood. While the title of the article stated that we were "Chipping Away at Breast Healthcare," the author was one Shaker Jane, "a proud abortioneer who is grateful every day for her Planned Parenthood and their work to protect reproductive rights."[5] This wasn't going to be about breast cancer care. It was going to be about abortion. And Planned Parenthood would sound the call to arms.

That night, at eight o'clock, someone tweeted that Komen had dropped Planned Parenthood. Another tweet went out at nine thirty the next morning. Both were sent prior to the Associated Press story's release.

Liz wrote the board Tuesday morning to let them know that Planned Parenthood had gone to the press and that the attack was about to begin. She gave an update on Nancy's call with Wasserman Schultz, saying that Wasserman Schultz had begged and badgered Nancy to continue supporting Planned Parenthood but that Nancy had stood firm. Liz also told the board members that the Associated Press piece would be coming out shortly, and that the reporter had spoken to Cecile before even picking up the phone to ask what was going on. Liz, sounding a bit frustrated to me, reiterated that the agreed-upon approach had been to do no proactive media, but that because the reporter had specific details of her private conversation with Cecile, a more detailed response was needed. She went on to say that this response was handled by Leslie—and me.

That was not true. Leslie did the on-the-record interview with Associated Press without my knowledge and despite Komen's statement-only strategy—one that Liz had reconfirmed that very afternoon. I believed that Leslie was simply getting background information from the reporter and had no idea that she would give an interview, let alone one focused on investigations instead of the approved press statement.

Liz advised the board that we were going to release the following statement: "As part of ongoing efforts to most effectively advance our mission, Komen is pursuing new strategies to allow for even greater investments in direct services for the women we serve and has implemented more stringent eligibility and performance criteria for our grants. While it is regrettable when changes in polices and strategic priorities affect any of our grantees, such as a longstanding partner like Planned Parenthood, we must continue to evolve our policies, programs, and strategies to best meet the needs of the women we serve and most fully advance our mission."

I felt then and believe to this day that Komen would have been far better off if we'd just stuck to the statement. Instead we were scrambling.

That day, frustrated beyond belief about everything—at myself mostly for not seeing that the sucker punch was coming, but also for not following Leslie to her office when she returned Associated Press's call, and at Hilary's gross misreading of the situation—I emailed Liz. I asked whether part of Hilary's role was to "calm the waters." I urged Liz that if it was, she needed to get Hilary into action. To my knowledge, nothing ever came of it.

Tsunami

The tidal wave itself hit on the afternoon of January 31. The *Huffington Post*—an admitted Planned Parenthood ally, and whose D.C. office is headed by the husband of Hilary's colleague Emily Lenzner—somehow had the Associated Press story before the news service had even posted it.

Very shortly after the *Huffington Post* piece appeared, the Associated Press story broke. Crary himself tweeted the story, with a link to the *Monterey County (Calif.) Herald*. The story was indeed a hit piece—of massive proportions. Crary led off by stating that we were halting our partnerships with Planned Parenthood, "creating a bitter rift, linked to the abortion debate, between two iconic organizations that have assisted millions of women."

The media made its play—the story would be focused on abortion and politics and not on the quality of the grants that Komen wanted to fund. The story didn't say a single word about grants and Komen's new strategy for them. The story trumpeted Planned Parenthood's claim that we ended grants because we had surrendered to "anti-abortion activists," and that according to Komen, "the key reason is that Planned Parenthood is under investigation in Congress—an inquiry launched by a conservative Republican who was urged to act by anti-abortion groups."

But the congressional investigation was *not* the key reason—it was never the key reason. I was distraught. I knew that we were now on the defensive.

At the same time, the story was media bias of the worst sort. If the story was going to focus on investigations, at least the reporter could have reported honestly and fully. Planned Parenthood wasn't under just one investigation—it was under multiple investigations in several different states. Second, the article omitted any mention of our new grant strategy—but perhaps that had not been mentioned in the interview. Further, the reporter used the term *anti-abortion* rather than *pro-life*. I don't think he would ever use the phrase *anti-life* to describe someone who is "pro-choice."

The story also quoted five people: Patrick Heard, CEO of Planned Parenthood of Southeastern Virginia, whose wife has breast cancer; Dottie Lamm, a fund-raiser for Planned Parenthood and wife of former Democratic Colorado governor Richard Lamm; Stephanie Kight, a vice president with Planned Parenthood of Orange and San Bernardino Counties; Leslie Aun; and Cecile Richards. Heard's quote was sufficiently heartbreaking: "We're kind of reeling. . . . It sounds almost trite, going through this with Betsi, but cancer doesn't care if you're pro-choice, anti-choice, progressive, conservative." The quote seemed to imply that Komen's funding to Planned Parenthood was related to treating women for breast cancer. This was not the case. Not a single grant to Planned Parenthood dealt with actually treating a woman with breast cancer.

Dottie Lamm's comments tugged even harder on the heart-strings: as a breast cancer survivor, she said, "It really makes me sad. . . . I kind of suspect there's a political agenda that got to Komen. . . . I hope it can be worked out."

Kight's comment was less emotional but just as effective. She said that both she and local Komen affiliates were frustrated with the situation.

Inexplicably, the comment attributed to Komen was that our main reason for cutting off the grants was the congressional investigation into Planned Parenthood. This was not true, and

Leslie had to know it wasn't true. Why would Leslie say that? Or perhaps she was misquoted? Regardless, we had now fallen right into Planned Parenthood's trap.

And Cecile was there to snap the trap shut. "It's hard to understand how an organization with which we share a mission of saving women's lives could have bowed to this kind of bullying," she said. "It's really hurtful." Cecile had actually used the word *bullying* just like the schoolyard tormenter says wide-eyed and innocently, "Who, me?" when caught in the act of beating up her classmate.

The piece rehashed Planned Parenthood press releases about the good the organization did. Cecile provided quotes that betrayed her private conversation with Liz. "It was incredibly surprising," she told Associated Press. "It wasn't even a conversation—it was an announcement."[6]

Planned Parenthood gladly accepted millions from Komen over the years. She and Liz—and Nancy, too—were supposedly friends. Planned Parenthood talked a good game about how we shared a mission—that both organizations worked to save women's lives. Yet Cecile was willing to cripple Komen over $680,000 in grants—less than one percent of Planned Parenthood's annual revenues. The reality is that Cecile was willing to sacrifice Komen's real work on behalf of women for raw political purposes that had nothing to do with serving women.

I now believe that Planned Parenthood relished the idea of bringing the situation into the open. They planned to do so all along. Blogs had the story before the story was out. Planned Parenthood supporters had their script before the story was out. The media, the Obama presidential campaign, and key Democrats followed the Planned Parenthood talking points and eagerly joined in to condemn Komen. Planned Parenthood linked up with MoveOn.org and Change.org. Key Democratic allies on the Hill already had statements and letters finalized and ready to go.

Planned Parenthood even leveraged Komen's demise for its own fund-raising. Within an hour or so after the Associated Press story was out, a Planned Parenthood mass email hit inboxes. Komen was the lead in its pitch for cash. "It's a deeply disappointing decision," read the email, "made even more alarming because politically motivated groups and individuals determined to undermine women's access to care appear to have successfully intimidated the Susan G. Komen for the Cure Foundation to withdraw this critical support." In short, they wrote, "right wing groups" had forced Komen out of association with "anti-choice groups."

"We know our opponents put their ideology over women's health and lives," Planned Parenthood sputtered. "What we never expected is that an ally like the Komen Foundation would choose to listen to them." These two sentences were bolded in the original email for emphasis. The email was signed by Cecile.

It was a gross mischaracterization. Cecile knew this. But she was the biggest bully of them all, smiling sweetly into the television camera as she deplored the actions that she claimed would leave women without breast health care—knowing that her statements were not true. She seemed happy to wield her club of outrage against Komen—the supposed friendship with Liz and the millions of dollars Komen had given to them over the years meant nothing. She appeared undaunted by the fact that her actions against Komen really would affect access to breast health care—the access that Komen provided through its other quality grants that actually made a difference.

But she wasn't the only bully. MoveOn.org joined the gang, sending its own fund-raising emails within minutes of the Associated Press story. The MoveOn.org email suggested that we had "bow[ed] to anti-choice pressure and [made] breast health care suddenly inaccessible to many women. . . . Without Komen's funding, many of these women could be unable to get the screenings and early detection of breast cancer that save lives. It's incredibly disappointing for an organization founded to protect women's health to play politics with real women's lives." They accused us of "joining the right-wing war on Planned Parenthood—which, let's be honest, is really a war on women." Taking a cue from the *Huffington Post,* they specifically targeted me, suggesting that I was Komen's link to "the anti-choice movement."

Despite the fact that I was not even mentioned in the Associated Press story, I was quickly becoming the focus of the ire of the blogosphere on the left. The *Huffington Post* kicked things off. And they did so with a scathing article about me. "The move comes less than a year after Komen hired a new vice president, who has publicly stated her opposition to abortion, a service provided at some Planned Parenthood facilities," *Huffington Post* leered. "Komen's new vice president, Karen Handel, had run for governor of Georgia in 2010 on an aggressively anti-abortion and anti–Planned Parenthood platform and was endorsed by Sarah Palin because of her opposition to reproductive choice. Handel wrote in her campaign blog that she 'do[es] not support the mission of Planned Parenthood.' "

This was outrageous. Yes, I am pro-life, and I did say I would work to defund Planned Parenthood in Georgia. But saying that I ran on an aggressive platform of these issues? I wasn't endorsed by a single pro-life organization. And it was well-known that Governor Palin and I did not share the exact same views on abortion. But that didn't stop the Planned Parenthood–friendly *Huffington Post* from plunging in the knife with a little guilt by association. In the minds of the left, because I was anti-abortion, I had sought out a position with Komen, had a plan, and somehow single-handedly persuaded Komen to adopt my nefarious anti–Planned Parenthood agenda.[7] How could anyone write this, let alone believe it? It was beyond absurd to think that I walked through the front door of Komen on April 4, 2011, and within months cast some kind of spell that convinced everyone to drop Planned Parenthood—as though I had some sort of supersecret pro-life powers. If I had had that kind of power, I would have become governor of Georgia, not a VP of public policy at Komen.

That didn't stop the *Huffington Post*.

The article received well over seven thousand comments.

———

Next came the *Jezebel* blog with its take: "Disgrace for the Cure." It garnered 137,000 Facebook likes. They, too, made me the focal point: "what accounts for the Komen Foundation's sudden change of heart? Surprisingly, it seems that the pressure may not have come from external sources, but from within the Foundation itself. . . . Last year's assault on Planned Parenthood also coincided with the addition of a vocally anti-abortion ex-politician to the ranks of Susan G. Komen for the Cure." Who was the person? Why, me, of course. "How curious!" *Jezebel* wrote. "A person with what looks like a personal vendetta against Planned Parenthood joins the ranks of an organization that provides funding to Planned Parenthood, and soon, that organization 'defunds' Planned Parenthood. But surely this couldn't be about Handel's personal feelings. According to Komen, this is about rule following. Protocol. If you believe that, I believe there's a bridge in Arizona you may be interested in buying."[8]

This was an all-out assault against Komen. We were being hit from every direction. I did not see coincidence; I saw coordination. It had to have been in the works for weeks—despite Hilary, who was hired specifically to "manage the left" and who told us that all was well. The "war on women" was on.

The Turmoil Begins

As soon as the Associated Press story was out, Katrina McGhee went on the offensive. I doubt she was really ever completely on board with the changes in the first place, even though she had indeed come to the conclusion that ending the Planned Parenthood grants was best for Komen—if for no other reason than for fund-raising. Now, with the blowback, she began to act.

After the Associated Press story broke over the wires, Katrina said that we had to move beyond our written statement. She said that she felt our strategy of statement-only was incomplete, but more than that, I got the sense that she wanted to reverse course. I didn't disagree totally with moving beyond the statement, now that we had already gotten ourselves completely off track. Maybe she was right—maybe we should have changed course at that point and immediately conducted in-depth interviews. I knew for certain that if we were explaining, we were losing. I argued that we needed to get back on message—talk about the high standards and excellence in grants. I also argued that putting Leslie back out for more press was a major risk, because she would be forced to address her comments to Associated Press. Who would do the interviews? Katrina wouldn't do it. I could do it, but I was obviously not the right person now that I was a target. And no one thought putting Liz or Nancy out there—at least at this time—was appropriate.

Katrina ensured that Nancy and the rest of us were up to speed on the negative response to the decision. She let us know that we had received just over two thousand complaints and only forty-six comments in support of the decision. I was not surprised by these numbers and said so. Planned Parenthood had orchestrated a broad email campaign that was enhanced by press releases, email blasts, and even TV news appearances by several Democratic members of Congress. I pointed out that I thought the response was more reflective of politics than anything to do with our mission.

Panic was beginning to set in among the executives at Komen.

By that night, it was obvious that Planned Parenthood was going for the kill. We were either with them—or dead. I recommended that we change course—fight back, as Liz had said we would do if Planned Parenthood chose an aggressive path. I suggested that we amend our statement to say something along the lines of "grant making decisions are not about politics—our priority is and always will be the women we serve. It is very disappointing that this issue has been leveraged for fundraising purposes and political gain." It seemed a perfectly reasonable statement and would turn the tables, at least calling into question Planned Parenthood's motives. It was vetoed.

Meanwhile, the talk on Twitter was now about me personally—and it was vicious. Apparently, although Leslie had not mentioned this to me or included it in her recap of her conversation with Associated Press, Crary had questioned her about my role at Komen, specifically asking if I was behind the decision. The *Huffington Post, Jezebel,* scores of other blogs, and thousands of tweets had made me the focus of their fury, using my personal political beliefs and a host of outright lies to make their case that I was the lone driver of the decision. Komen's social media manager (who I would learn was out most of the week) advised Liz and Nancy of the situation. Twitter was slamming me for running a supposed anti–Planned Parenthood gubernatorial campaign and now I was head of Komen's public policy, hammering the notion that my personal beliefs were a factor in Komen's policy decisions. Oddly, I was not directly copied on that email. Liz would eventually forward it to me.

My husband would later look at my Twitter followers. What

he found was interesting. I had been on somebody's radar screen for months. My Twitter followers had been stable for months. Then in December, the number of followers jumped significantly, from fewer than 2,500 in mid-December to about 3,100 by the end of January. It was a sudden and dramatic spike—a 24 percent increase—for no reason. After the Associated Press and *Huffington Post* stories, someone hacked my Twitter account—not Anthony Weiner–style, but for real. First, they tweeted something about a Komen race. There was just one problem: the race they referenced didn't exist. Then the hacker retweeted an anti–Planned Parenthood message: "Just like a pro-abortion group to turn a cancer orgs decision into a political bomb to throw. Cry me a freaking river." It was first reported by an anonymous source on the MoveOn.org website. A click on the link took you to an individual with Fund Abortion Now.

A fake Facebook page was set up next. Maudlin messages were posted in my name. "As I told the NY Times," read one, "please respect my right to privacy at this difficult time. You people hurt my feelings." The commenters were just as nasty as the hacker. "Skank," wrote one. The person wrote back in my name, "Eat s*** and die, you PAGAN WHORE!!" And "Send money!!"

Trying to Cope

On Wednesday morning, early, I touched based with Nancy and Liz. Planned Parenthood had clearly deceived us, and their attack had been in the making for some time, I asserted. To me, the sympathetic reporter, a fund-raising email primed and ready, the timing of the Wasserman Schultz call, help from the Daily Kos website and other liberal outfits that were not only lined up but already briefed—all pointed to premeditation, even as Planned Parenthood was leading Komen on. I floated the idea that now we probably needed to start identifying allies for Komen. Planned Parenthood had made our original desire of "no scalp for either side" impossible. We had not lined up allies or secured third-party advocates at this point. The reason: we had been keeping our promise to Planned Parenthood not to make a public scene over the decision, and word that we were proactively lining up support would have almost certainly made its way to the press and back to Planned Parenthood.

Nancy expressed her frustration about the situation. She was offended and disturbed by Planned Parenthood's lack of professionalism and their tactics. I thought I sensed a note of true sadness when she said that her parents had told her about evil and that she had never really believed it or that it would come from a group that Komen had helped so much.

All I could tell Liz and Nancy—who were both clearly distraught—was to hang in there.

I wanted to be sure that Nancy and Liz received the full picture of our situation—the bad but also the good, because there were those who supported Komen's actions. I began forwarding some of the positive emails to them.

By this time, the team from Ogilvy was in the Komen offices. If Hilary and Leslie were in touch, Leslie had not passed along any update. Neither Nancy nor Liz mentioned that they'd heard from Hilary, and generally, they would have given the team an update if Hilary had provided any guidance. I was perplexed that, in this time of crisis, Hilary appeared to be unengaged.

That morning, we finally heard from SKDKnickerbocker when someone from the firm sent over a redraft of our press statement. But by this time, Katrina, Brendan, Leslie, and Morris + King (one of Komen's other PR firms) were focused on Nancy doing limited on-air interviews. Hilary next provided a list of key statements that she suggested we send to various pro-choice organizations. She provided an Excel spreadsheet that listed about twenty or thirty organizations, but most of the contact information was missing. I wasn't sure how this was supposed to help and whether Hilary expected us to divert our focus in the middle of a crisis to track down information for her contact list.

The statements she proposed struck me as off base. Hilary suggested that we tell these pro-choice groups that Komen had no interest in a public fight with Planned Parenthood, that Komen supported Planned Parenthood's mission, and that we were still funding them. She also wanted us to say that Planned Parenthood had two clinics in the United States that offered direct breast screening services and that Komen was funding them. The only problem with this last sentence was that there were no Planned Parenthood clinics that provided mammograms directly.

Meanwhile, Brendan Daly and others from Ogilvy had set up a crisis war room in the Komen offices. While Brendan Daly and Leslie had sketched out a good outline of a crisis communications plan at the end of 2011, it seemed as though there had been little follow-through. But they were working diligently on several different angles: a formal Facebook note from Nancy, an

FAQ Facebook note, a short video from Brinker to be posted on YouTube, etc.

Nancy would go with the idea of a video for YouTube. It was called "Straight Talk." It was a complete bust. People saw it as contrived and forced. And they were right.

When it came to social media, Komen was completely out-flanked. Some took Komen to task for not being more prepared and engaged when it came to social media. I would ask everyone to consider that Komen is a breast cancer organization; it is fo-cused on ending breast cancer. Moreover, it was already mindful of the need to transition from the small nonprofit mentality to more sophisticated approaches. Komen was in the process of do-ing just that, with its grants strategy—for which it was now being pummeled—and in various other areas, including communica-tions, social media, and even marketing and fundraising.[9]

To a great degree, Planned Parenthood's sophisticated online campaign, coupled with the efforts of other groups equally as so-cial media savvy, was a major success factor. But let's also remem-ber that Planned Parenthood is a veteran at guerrilla grassroots warfare, having built an army of true believers ready to do battle whenever Cecile issues the call—whether to attack a breast can-cer organization or to help elect Planned Parenthood's candidates of choice.

Twitter and Facebook exploded in a coordinated attack on behalf of Planned Parenthood. Within minutes of the story breaking, both were swamped with pro–Planned Parenthood, anti-Komen messages. The ratio of anti-Komen to pro-Komen tweets was reaching epic proportions—80 to 1. Energizer, one of our corporate sponsors, began receiving wall posts threatening a boycott until Komen reengaged with Planned Parenthood. Secondary boycotts had become the domain of the left—they'd used them against Don Imus and Glenn Beck and would later employ the tactic against Rush Limbaugh and the American Legislative Exchange Council. Now these same bullies were testing the maneuver on Komen.

Katrina was pushing us to release a full list of investigations into Planned Parenthood. We had the list, but I thought getting mired in these details was a mistake. I still believed that our mission was our best message.

We were floundering so much that Liz and Nancy seemed unsure about the counsel they were getting from Komen executives and existing consultants. They began contacting others and bringing in even more advisors. By this time I was beginning to be cut out of the loop—no doubt thanks to the Associated Press and the *Huffington Post*. I was toxic material.

Cecile was continuing to take full advantage. One of our people made a five-dollar donation to Planned Parenthood to keep track of Planned Parenthood's anti-Komen propaganda. A robo-response from Cecile was almost immediate and included a request to sign the following petition: "This is for all the anti-choice, anti-women people out there. Listen up. You can spend every minute of every day trying to force the rest of us to live by your ideology. You can go after federal funds for health care and pressure private organizations like the Susan G. Komen for the Cure Foundation to stop funding breast cancer screenings for poor women. You can try to make it impossible to get birth control. But you know what you can't do? You can't win. You can't break us. . . . Know this: When you go after Planned Parenthood and the people they serve, you go after ME." Cecile noted, "I signed that open letter with pride, because it captures exactly how I feel."

The hypocrisy of the email reached new heights—even for Cecile. Cecile and Planned Parenthood were complaining that pro-life forces were targeting "private organizations." Yet wasn't that what Planned Parenthood was doing? Cecile and Planned Parenthood were screaming that pro-life forces were spending "every minute of every day trying to force the rest of us to live by [their] ideology." And yet here was Planned Parenthood trying to drive us into their ideological camp by subjecting us to severe public pressure and private backstabbing. Komen wanted no part of either side. We wanted to be neutral—free to be focused on one thing: ending breast cancer forever.

Members of Congress—the Democrats—also weighed in. Amazingly, less than twenty-four hours after the Associated Press story, Congressman Mike Honda (D-CA) distributed a "Dear Colleague" letter asking members to join him in signing a letter to Komen urging a reversal—that letter was already drafted. A similar effort was under way in the U.S. Senate. This seemed an amazing accomplishment—not because senators sent a letter, but because of how quickly the letter came. It was a lightning-fast turnaround—just forty-eight hours to get staff sign-off on content and secure the signatures from more than two dozen members.

Despite all of that, there were some signs that the tide was turning a bit with general public opinion. Leslie informed us that evening that we'd received 33,000 emails—and that positive emails were now outpacing the negative by a ratio of 2 to 1. Nancy was cautiously optimistic. Katrina was less so and said that there was no way to know what any of this meant until we compared it to our donor base. She had had no such reservations the day before when the email count heavily favored Planned Parenthood.

Later that night, I emailed the executive team to share what I thought was more encouraging news. More than one thousand people had signed a petition supporting Komen's decision on Planned Parenthood. Katrina responded that, while she was glad there were some positive people, it wasn't good enough, because these people, she said, were not supporting Komen's mission. Rather they were supporting a decision that they considered anti-abortion.

I was perplexed by her comments. Why was she responding in such a negative way? Just as we didn't know if the positive emails were Komen donors, we didn't know if the negative emailers were donors, either. Also, why were the motives of those who supported the decision now so relevant? The individuals berating Komen because of the decision certainly weren't concerned with our mission—they were angry because they saw this as anti-abortion and anti–Planned Parenthood.

The Big Mistake

All we had to do was play prevent defense. We were receiving more and more emails expressing support for the decision.

The storm seemed to be abating. Unfortunately, the panic had already spread too deep.

Katrina and others had now convinced Liz and Nancy that we had to get on the TV news shows. Komen's media consultants in New York, Morris + King, had been recommending this, too. Brendan Daly, from Ogilvy, was also on board with this play—as was Leslie. We were all informed on Wednesday morning that the decision had been made. Komen would do one interview with what was called a "friendly reporter." It was decided that the friendly reporter was Andrea Mitchell. Katrina directed Morris + King to pursue the interview and ensure that it could take place the next day. The interview would be one-on-one— just Mitchell and Komen; there would be no point/counterpoint exchanges.

I still thought that our best course was to just let Planned Parenthood and the left wail away. This story would eventually give way to a new one. The Super Bowl was Sunday, and the game, along with other news, would eventually take over. And I didn't believe there was any such thing as a "friendly reporter."

But Komen had some of the most experienced communications professionals on retainer, so I supposed they must be right—and I began to consider that this might be an opportunity.

It was still unclear who would actually do the interview. Liz was now in Washington but Nancy was still in Florida. Finally, it was decided that Nancy had to do the interview, but she would do it from Florida—remotely. That was a horrible idea. Doing the interview remotely would put Nancy at a real disadvantage, making a difficult interview all the more so. Next, someone suggested that Nancy and Liz do the interview together. Another awful idea. Finally, Nancy decided to travel to D.C. immediately in order to do the interview live and in person.

Meanwhile, the *New York Times* and others were clamoring for interviews.

I now had some time on my hands. I thought more about the Mitchell interview and various scenarios for how it might go. The more I thought about it, the less I liked the idea.

Katrina and Nancy and Liz—with Morris + King, Brendan, and Leslie—had decided on Mitchell not because she was on our side—she was anything but. They settled on her because she was a breast cancer survivor and Nancy's friend. They didn't just think Mitchell was a good option for the interview—they thought she was *perfect*.

Everyone knew the interview was important. So Liz and company called a meeting of the "murder board."

Little did they know how apt the term would be.

8

Implosion

On Thursday morning, February 2, 2012, in Washington, D.C., the Komen conference room was packed as the "murder board" was called to order. Twelve people sat around a table—with more on the phone—all gathered to grill Nancy in preparation for her interview with Andrea Mitchell later that morning.

The murder board was a committee of individuals brought together to run Nancy through a rigorous role-play focusing on anticipated questions from Mitchell. The U.S. military originally came up with the phrase.[1] It's an effective tool—when done right. But rather than prepare Nancy to survive a possibly deadly interview, it would be a death nail—quite literally an omen of destruction combined with the proverbial nail in the coffin.

Ogilvy's Brendan Daly was the meeting leader. I was there—I had not been totally shut out yet. A who's who of D.C.'s most prominent communications and crisis management experts had been assembled. Komen's murder board members were Brad Blakeman, a former George W. Bush appointee and frequent network news political analyst; Mark Dybul, also a former Bush appointee, and the lead on the president's Emergency Plan for

AIDS Relief—he was there because he had experience in facing off with Planned Parenthood; Mason Essif, former CNN and ABC journalist now with Ogilvy; another crisis communications expert whom Komen had previously attempted to hire; two or three other Ogilvy staffers; and John Raffaelli, a Komen board member and prominent lobbyist with strong Democratic ties—he had worked for the late senator Lloyd Bentsen (D-TX), served on the Clinton-Gore finance committee, and been vice chair of John Kerry's presidential campaign. Also in the room were Leslie Aun, Komen consultant Brian Hook, Liz Thompson, and, of course, Nancy Brinker.

On the phone we had Judith King and Caren Browning with Morris + King, Nancy's son Eric Brinker, and Komen policy consultant Rae Evans.

Hilary Rosen was not in the meeting or on the phone. I thought it extremely odd, given the role she had been specifically hired to fill.

As we got started, I recalled something that my friend Dan McLagan, who was the communications director for my governor's campaign, would say: "Everybody has their turn at the bottom of the barrel." Komen was having its turn, and we simply had to persevere—to push through it. With the weekend and the Super Bowl game—and the likelihood of the next big story—the press would move on. And even if they didn't, we knew that the tenor of the debate would start to shift. Those on the other side were beginning to weigh in. Cooler heads were pointing out that Komen had the right to make whatever decision it wanted for its organization.

I believed that what was most important—indeed critical—at

this juncture and with the Mitchell interview was to do nothing that would create new news. We had to avoid lighting a spark that could reignite the firestorm. If we could get to Friday, I was convinced that things would begin to die down.

———

My sense of dread grew as the meeting progressed. Nancy seemed visibly shaken.

The only thing anyone had agreed on was the fact that the interview would be fifteen minutes, live. The debate on what to actually say went in circles. Some even reopened the discussion of who would do the interview. Perhaps Nancy should not do it, given her politics?

The murder board session was complete pandemonium—more of an exercise in futility than a professional preparatory session for an important interview.

Although Liz was present, she was focused on her Black-Berry. I wasn't able to get her attention, so I sent an email. I expressed my serious concerns about the meeting. Input and counsel from broad perspectives was appropriate and beneficial, but with so many people, the session would quickly turn to chaos. I told Liz that she and Nancy would need some quiet time before heading to the studio and that there wasn't time to keep rehashing the same points. I pointed out that she and Nancy had to be comfortable with the direction; that Nancy's ability to come across as confident and genuine was key. Liz never responded. I kept wondering what could have been more important than what was happening in that room at that moment.

Everyone talked at once—shouting out ideas; drowning out

others. Issues that had already been settled were rehashed. For example, it was already decided that Nancy would do the interview. Mitchell was expecting her. Yet time was spent debating whether Nancy's politics (I assumed because she was a Republican) made her less than ideal. Finally, the group settled on a few points: be consistent on our position regarding the investigations; convey that Komen's community support was not being reduced—that, in fact, the Planned Parenthood dollars were being directed to better purposes—and emphasize that there would be no gap in care for indigent women. In short, the very points that should have been made in that first interview with Associated Press.

Brendan Daly was an expert in communications and crisis management, as were others in the room. But I was surprised by the way the meeting was conducted. I thought I had never been in one that was more chaotic, and less focused.

In the midst of the madness, one important topic was glossed over: me. I had a list of tough questions that included "What about your politics?" and "What about KCH?" While I had been invited to attend the meeting, by this time there was little interest in my counsel or thoughts. It seemed to me that Nancy headed to her interview dazed and unsure. My sense of dread worsened. With any murder board, someone was usually left for dead. It just had not fully sunk in that that person would be me.

The Ambush

The interview with Nancy and Mitchell was a fiasco—from word one. Mitchell attacked—she pounced on Nancy and quickly made me the focus. Mitchell seemed to have her briefing paper from Planned Parenthood and *Huffington Post*, going through the items point by point. Nancy did her best, but it was not enough. She seemed timid and uncertain—no doubt thanks, in large part, to the thoroughly inadequate and unfocused prep she had received. Here's the transcript of the interview, in relevant part:

MITCHELL: Ambassador Nancy Brinker is the founder and CEO of Susan G. Komen for the Cure and joins me now.

Well, the storm has exploded, and you've been in this for a long time. You started Susan G. Komen in 1982 after the death of your sister and in her name. And you have raised more money than any other group for breast cancer research.

Which is why I have to tell you this is shocking for a lot of your longtime supporters. I want to give you a chance to answer—let me just tell you what I was confronted with at the gym this morning. A woman came over to me, I had not met her before, gray-haired woman, probably in her sixties, she was wearing a gray T-shirt, and she said, "Look at my T-shirt. It's inside out. I put it on by accident today. I'm not going to wear it anymore. I've torn the label out. It's a Komen T-shirt."

These are longtime supporters who have run with you, who have supported you financially and otherwise. So they're asking, how could this have taken place?

BRINKER: Well, Andrea, I frankly think, I don't know, it's a mischaracterization, of certainly, of our goals, our mission, and everything that we do. In fact, we haven't defunded Planned

Parenthood. We still have three grants that we've committed to, at least for another year, through the end of the grant cycle, and we're going to—

MITCHELL: But that's just through the end of the grant cycle. Let me just put out there first of all, that I have been very identified, an outspoken supporter and participant in the races over the years long before I, myself, ended up being diagnosed with breast cancer. So I want to just put that out there. We've known each other a long time as well, both when you were a diplomat at the State Department.

But I come to you today, you know, expressing the anger of a lot of people—

"Expressing the anger" of people? This was completely inappropriate. Mitchell was a journalist. Why was it her job to "express the anger" of people? Wasn't her job to report—with at least some degree of impartiality? It was a hit job, pure and simple—executed by a member of the Planned Parenthood mafia. Mitchell would later praise Planned Parenthood as a noble organization.[2]

BRINKER: Sure.

MITCHELL: Channeling through them, you see it on Twitter, you see it everywhere. And the fact is, a lot of people are tracing this back. My colleague, Lisa Myers, reporting last night on *Nightly News*, a lot of people are tracing this back to what some found the surprising hiring of Karen Handel, who ran for governor. We've seen her statements and her strong support. She said

when she was running for office, "I am staunchly and unequivocally pro-life. Let me be clear, since I am pro-life, I do not support the mission of Planned Parenthood."

So, the question is, for a bipartisan organization such as
yours, which has a broad-based advisory group, why hire a key
staff person who is so strongly, fiercely identified against Planned
Parenthood, one of your grantees?

The response was simple: Komen *is* a bipartisan organization,
and as such, we had to reach out to people on both sides of the
political aisle. That's why I had been hired. Mitchell suggested
that hiring someone who is Republican or pro-life somehow
broke an unwritten rule and that no one with these beliefs should
be allowed to work for Komen. That was absurd. Unfortunately,
Nancy fell right into the trap:

BRINKER: Well, let me just for the record tell you, Karen did not
have anything to do with this decision. This was decided at the
board level and also by our mission, Andrea. Everything that we
get up and do every day is about the mission. To provide women,
vulnerable populations, with care, treatment, and screening.

Oh no. This was not true. I *was* part of the decision-making
process. This was obvious from my title. By going so far in deny-
ing my involvement, Nancy had inadvertently just made the new
news that I had worried so much about—this would certainly
keep this story alive. The left and the blogs would immediately
jump on Nancy's statement as a "lie." I didn't think Nancy was

being deceptive. I thought she was trying to be protective of me and to convey that, as CEO, the buck stopped with her.

BRINKER: And let me just take a step back for a minute. We are not defunding Planned Parenthood. We have three grants that will go on this year, and they will probably be eligible for the next grant cycle—

MITCHELL: But you've said that this is the one group out of two thousand grantees, Planned Parenthood is the only group that comes under the rubric of this new policy, which is to not fund any organization that is under investigation. And their investigation, from Congressman [Cliff] Stearns [R-FL], many believe is trumped up.

Mitchell was putting words in Nancy's mouth. We never said this. Even Leslie, in her off-message statements, had not said this. We had new policies, plural, and we expected numerous organizations to be affected one way or the other. A large hospital in a major metropolitan city was affected by the more stringent eligibility criteria. While we never said it publicly, out of what I believe was seriously misguided respect for the longtime partnership, Komen should have already rescinded Planned Parenthood's grants based on previous precedent. As we demanded more meaningful outcomes, crappy grants—like those with Planned Parenthood—would no longer measure up. We would invest our dollars for the biggest impact. When Nancy tried to answer, Mitchell talked over her—a steamroller. Nancy, usually assertive and in control, lost control of the interview. When I finally watched the entire interview, nothing was more personally frustrating to me than this segment:

BRINKER: Well, but there are other investigations in states, number one. Two—

MITCHELL: They're always the target of an investigation. That's the way—

BRINKER: The investigation isn't the only issue, Andrea. In 2010, we set about creating excellence in our grants. Not just in our community grants, but in our science grants. Putting metrics, outcomes, and measures to them so that we can translate all of the science we funded over thirty years.

Now, part of that includes taking these grants into communities and being excellent grant givers. Many of the grants we were doing with Planned Parenthood do not meet new standards of criteria for how we can measure our results and effectiveness in communities. That is not to say that if they did meet those criteria, they would not be—

MITCHELL: Their supporters say they are the only ones that have been singled out among these thousands—

BRINKER: No, that's not true. That's not true.

MITCHELL: —and that their grants for breast screening have nothing to do with any contraceptive or abortion counseling.

BRINKER: It's not—

MITCHELL: That they separate this funding completely.

BRINKER: The issue—that's not the issue. Because that's not our issue. Our issue is grant excellence. They do pass-through grants with their screening grants. They send people to other facilities.

We want to do more direct-service grants. You know, we contacted them in the fall, because we've been a longtime partner of Planned Parenthood, almost twenty years.

MITCHELL: I know.

BRINKER: We've given them over nine million dollars. Many of our grants worked for a long period of time.

This is not—this is about the restructure of our grant program. Now, as an NGO and as a leader in the breast cancer space, we have an obligation to the community we serve, to donors, and to this country to translate cancer care in the way we know how.

Mitchell said she "knew" that Komen had contacted Planned Parenthood months ago. How did she know? But at least, Nancy finally seemed to be getting her bearings. Mitchell appeared to be deliberately ignoring the points Nancy was making, and instead—on national television—made what sounded a lot to me like a threat of lost financial resources. The power of the media was now brought to bear directly on Komen. Mitchell had traded her journalistic code of ethics for a role as the emissary of the Obama administration, of Planned Parenthood, and, more generally, of the left. This was Mitchell's *Godfather* moment. "Nice foundation you've got there," she seemed to be saying. "Shame if something happened to it."

MITCHELL: What do you do about the fact that donors are pulling back? Some people would say that—I mean, the anger that's being expressed is going to hit you in the pocketbook. You have worked so hard to create a bipartisan organization. Look at your Facebook page. Your Facebook page has people cutting pink ribbons in half.

BRINKER: Well, Andrea—

MITCHELL: Your branding is at stake.

BRINKER: —all I can tell you is that the responses we're getting are very, very favorable. People who have bothered to read the material, who have bothered to understand the issues—again, we work for a mission, every day of our lives. And our job now is to translate cancer therapy into usable types of therapies that can be accessible for people—

It was as though Mitchell was executing Planned Parenthood's game plan—play by play. She portrayed Komen as a politically motivated organization determined to deprive needy women of their vital health care.

MITCHELL: Aren't the most vulnerable women going to be affected by this? Planned Parenthood—

BRINKER: We are not giving less money in the communities where we're giving money. Let me just set the record straight: where we are giving money in these communities, we are not taking it back. We will, with some of them, go to direct service providers.

But we still have these grants in place with Planned Parenthood, in places where there aren't direct service providers, and they are good grants and they work with us.

But unless we have a way, again, to measure grants, to create metrics, outcomes in ways that we can say, this works in this community with this vulnerable population, this is what will work. These are the barriers, this is how it works. That is our only mission, to cure breast cancer.

Nancy was beginning to make her points. But Mitchell wasn't done. Now she wanted Komen to make public internal records regarding the Planned Parenthood grants. Komen was a private organization with the right to set whatever policies it deemed necessary and in its best interest. Besides, the issue was not the quality of Planned Parenthood's work. We were not saying that Planned Parenthood wasn't a good provider. We were simply saying that it wasn't the best provider for what we wanted to accomplish going forward.

MITCHELL: Are you going to put out the evidence that you have that there's been anything flawed in the way they've delivered services to—

BRINKER: All we're doing is explaining, again, to our mission, what the criteria for new grants and community-based grants are, for our organization, for the time we are.

Many of the grants were education-oriented. We don't need to do that kind of education anymore. We've done it for thirty years. Now we need to translate this care into usable clinical care in communities. That means that if a person's screened, we need to follow. We need to follow up the screening. Did something happen. Once they go through the Planned Parenthood program, they also have to come to us for additional therapy and care.

We are trying to advise our community grant program. And we're doing it, and they've been a longtime partner of ours. We've notified them of this change, and frankly, we've been very private about it. And we have not said that we won't accept grants who meet our criteria.

MITCHELL: Ambassador Nancy Brinker, thank you very much.

BRINKER: Thanks, Andrea.

The interview was a complete disaster—far worse than I could have imagined. By Thursday afternoon, I was out of the loop on all things strategic. I wasn't sure if this was at the direction of Nancy or Liz or not. They had not said anything to me. Meetings continued well into the night.

A Firestorm Reignited

The biggest mistake of the interview was clearly Nancy's statement that I had nothing to do with the decision. The comment and our evolving messages made it seem like Komen was trying to hide something. Saying that I had nothing to do with the decision, when it was obvious that I was involved, intensified the attention on me and fueled the ridiculous argument that I was some kind of pro-life Trojan horse. Blogs were calling Nancy a liar. I was the senior vice president of public policy—how could I have had nothing to do with it? Again, I don't think Nancy was trying to be deceptive. She took her leadership responsibilities to heart. But in saying what she said, she fed the media beast—and instigated a fresh assault from the liberal army.

As soon as the interview ended, the new offensive was launched—nasty emails and phones call started. They were largely directed at me personally. "You are a disgrace to women and you should not only lose your role at the Komen Foundation but you should be shut out of any organization with a mission to help others, especially women or children," wrote one emailer. "Shame on you for letting your political views guide you in such a detrimental way to women. You make me sick." The meanness continued—becoming harsher and more vicious throughout the day. Later that afternoon, our website was attacked.

The mail wasn't all one-sided, of course. Some people emailed to thank me personally. I found these emails just as puzzling—I was just one person who had obviously not acted unilaterally. I was part of the team. It was the media that portrayed me as mastermind of the Komen–Planned Parenthood breakup.

In the office, the mood continued to shift—the initial stand-our-ground toughness evolved into panic, which was followed by cautious optimism as Nancy headed to the Mitchell interview. That cautious optimism had now faded, and I could sense the resolve weakening. Everyone tried to put a good face on the Mitchell interview, but there was a feeling that we were in serious trouble.

Somebody hacked the Twitter feed of Jill Biden, wife of Vice President Joe Biden, and put out a message: "When Joe heard about Susan G. Komen not funding Planned Parenthood anymore, Joe threw away his pink-ribbon Harvest Peach yogurt." The media quickly reported it as a real tweet. Liberal politicians across the country now saw their opportunity and were joining in to condemn Komen.

Katrina was wondering where all the vocal support was from the conservative side of the aisle. Nancy was wondering this, too. I reminded everyone that Komen had agreed to "a scalp for neither side." We had purposely held back the applause from conservatives. We had been very careful in the run-up to the decision and afterward to do all we could to ensure that conservatives were not doing happy dances in the street. I had done the job I was tasked to do; the same could not be said for those who were supposed to manage the left.

Unlike Planned Parenthood, we did not have letters from Congress teed up. We had not lined up a parade of surrogates, prepped and ready to fight. We purposely did not mobilize pro-life organizations in our own defense. We could easily have done all that. But Komen meant what Liz said to Cecile Richards—there was no desire to create another issue for them; our decision was not based on the politics of abortion. We kept our word, true to our desire to give a "scalp to neither side."

Some assumed we were simply unprepared. We were prepared—prepared to manage a disagreement about how to best deliver breast health services. We were not prepared for an attack by a seasoned, cold-blooded political entity on the battle-field of abortion politics in an election fight for the hearts—and votes—of women.

It was a near-fatal mistake. We were outgunned and overwhelmed. Heck, we didn't even put up a fight. I should have factored in Nancy's susceptibility to public opinion and pushed harder for a more aggressive posture. But more importantly, I should have known that Planned Parenthood would respond *politically*—not altruistically. I should have anticipated that

they—Planned Parenthood and the left—would use our decision
in the broader political war being waged. Ironically, by keeping politics out of our decision, we overlooked the raw political
aspects of the issue and failed to consider politics as a factor. We
believed that our reputation as global leaders in breast cancer
would sustain us—we had always put our mission first. This was
no different.

Many Komen affiliates were in open mutiny. Some were
even coordinating with Planned Parenthood and threatening
to walk away from Komen. This was little more than a paper
threat in terms of the practicality of actually carrying it out, but
it created more panic within Komen. Several affiliates even told
the press they had no idea that the decision was coming. This
was simply not the case, because there had been scores of calls
with individual affiliates leading up to the January 1 effective
date, and the affiliates were well aware of Komen's outcomes-
based granting strategy. It had been under way since 2010, but
I suppose that some didn't think through the actual implica-
tions of the strategy. CBS in Los Angeles reported that our
Los Angeles affiliate executive director had resigned because of
Planned Parenthood. This was not true. She had resigned earlier
and Liz confirmed to the press that her resignation had been
unrelated.[3]

Some of the same affiliates that cheered the new direction,
relieved that they could finally move on from the Planned Parenthood controversies, were now turning against us, too. While
the local pressure was intense on the affiliates, I suspected that
the affiliates leading the charge were doing so for reasons unre-

lated to their commitment to Komen's mission. The angriest affiliates were those with the strongest ties to Planned Parenthood.
These were some of the same affiliate staffers who, at the Komen
affiliates meeting the previous July, stated vehemently that protecting a woman's right to choose trumped Komen's mission to
end breast cancer, even if Komen had to suffer. Many of the affiliates threatening to walk were the very same affiliates who had
been most vocal about the proposed restructuring that would reduce the number of affiliates and fold those that remained into a
single organization. It seemed to me that these affiliates had just
found a way to hold Komen National as a hostage for demands of
their own.

Komen was being torn apart—enemies we didn't even know we
had were joining forces. Despondency was palpable throughout
the office. Brendan had been around our offices all day February 1 and 2, managing communications with Leslie. At one
point he wandered into my office, sat down, and sighed in defeat,
"What a mess."

Thursday night, I learned that John Raffaelli, a board member
and Planned Parenthood backer, had an idea—one that I thought
was rather strange. He would reach out to Senator Frank Lauten-
berg (D-NJ) and broker a compromise based on Komen adding
the word *criminal* to the grant criteria regarding investigations.
Inserting the word *criminal* would put Planned Parenthood back
in good standing, Raffaelli and others reasoned. In fact, adding
criminal would actually make things worse for Planned Parent-

hood, since many of the investigations into Planned Parenthood *were* criminal, involving allegations of Medicaid fraud, sex trafficking, and illegal abortions, such as underage and late-term. Now, there were even allegations that Planned Parenthood was facilitating sex-selection abortions. There were even formal indictments—felony and misdemeanor—that had been handed down by a county grand jury in Kansas.

It was complete chaos.

Then the bomb threats and suspicious packages started. Truly sick people were threatening me with bodily harm.

At the same time, Planned Parenthood and its pals turned their fury on our corporate sponsors. Our sponsors were scared—they'd seen what the Democratic machine could do when it decided on a target for destruction. They were right to be frightened. But some stuck with us openly. RE/MAX issued a statement, explaining that "because we feel that Komen is making a real difference in women's lives, we have made the decision to maintain our sponsorship of the national Susan G. Komen Race for the Cure. Because we know that Komen does not make funding and policy decisions based on political considerations, we are confident that our support of this organization is in the best interest of all women. While they have changed their partnership program policies, Komen is not canceling grants but is creating a new, forward-looking grant policy."

The calls for my resignation were growing. There were hundreds of emails and phones calls, and petitions circulating the Internet that had already garnered thousands of signatures. The left had taken a page directly out of the Saul Alinsky playbook:

pick the target, freeze it, personalize it, polarize it. They needed someone to demonize—and that someone was me.

Capitulation

Desperation permeated the office.

But oddly, the facts didn't support the despair. By Thursday afternoon, February 2, despite the disastrous Andrea Mitchell interview, things were beginning to move on a better course.

Since Tuesday, when the initial Associated Press story hit, Komen's online donations had doubled from the previous year, and *increased* as the week went on. At one point, Komen's number of single-day contributors had increased 200 percent versus the prior year, and donations were up 400 percent.

The tenor of emails was shifting, too. We'd received more than 125,000 emails. They were running nearly 50,000 in support of the decision and just over 17,000 against. Even with the 50,000 or so that still had to be sorted, this was at least a bit of good news. But Katrina continued to insist that we had to be judicious with this information and refrain from reading into the emails a surge of support.

I got to the office early on Friday morning. When I checked my email, I learned that Liz had done a press roundtable the day before in which she'd told reporters that investigations had nothing to do with the decision.[4] This wasn't exactly true, either. The investigations certainly weren't the sole reason or even the primary reason, but they were *a* reason, because stricter rules had been put in place to drive the quality of the grants and the grantees. I was at a loss, especially since it was Liz herself who pointed out Komen's past precedent for revoking grants based on investigations, citing the Mississippi Health Department investigation. But far more damaging was that Komen's message had changed yet again, and this was a complete reversal of what Nancy had said.

This would start an entirely new round of questions. With so many different responses, Komen had now made it nearly impossible for anyone to understand what we did or why.

The next morning, I ran into Liz in the small break room, and we had a short conversation:

"How are you?" she asked.

"I'm fine."

"Well," she said, sighing, "this is an absolute disaster. We're having a meeting this morning, and we have to decide what we're going to do. I think we're going to reinstate their eligibility. We have no choice."

I wasn't surprised, but I had to give my candid counsel. "That would be a monumental mistake, Liz," I said. "If we just stick this out—"

She cut me off, saying, "This is no longer about ideology."

This had *never* been about ideology, and Liz knew it. I was not going to let Liz or anyone else suggest that it was.

"Let's be abundantly clear," I said. "Liz, you know and I know that this was never about ideology. How dare you make that statement to me." And then I added, "As you have your meetings," I continued, "you'd better get your arms around the leak within Komen. There's a gigantic sieve in this organization, and it's going right to Planned Parenthood and outlets like *Huffington Post*."

I had no idea who the leaker was, but I knew it was detrimental to Komen.

At that point Liz had to go to her meeting. I knew that the board was rattled.

Sure enough, later that morning, Liz and Nancy both walked into my office. "We're so sorry," said Nancy. "We're so sorry. But we just have to reverse course."

I just said, "You don't have to apologize to me. But I have to say again that it is a huge mistake. Wait through the weekend. It's Super Bowl weekend. We know there are op-eds teed up about how outrageous Planned Parenthood is being, that private organizations have the right to make the decisions they believe are best. If we blink now, it's over and no one will know what Komen stands for," I implored.

Nancy's reply stunned me. "Karen, I've talked to a lot of people. And even Karl says we have to backtrack. There's just no other way."

"Karl? Who's Karl?"

She looked at me strangely as if I should know exactly who she was talking about. She said, "Karl Rove!"

I started laughing. Just when I thought things could not get more bizarre. What in the world did Karl Rove have to do with anything?

Nancy continued. "This is the only way," she reiterated. "You have no idea what I've been through over the past three days."

Nancy sank down in her chair, shaking her head and rubbing her face as she does sometimes. She and Liz kept going on and on about how they had no choice, apologizing and talking about leadership. I had stopped listening.

I was upset, disappointed, and angry. I was disappointed that Komen was refusing to fight for our mission. I was angry about the lies and distortions that were playing out in the media and on blogs and Twitter. I had been a professional and had done my job in Komen's best interest. I had never wanted to be in the middle of this issue, and now I was being thrown under the bus as a result of it.

We anticipated a significant backlash. To be sure, we did not anticipate this playing out in such a political way, but we all knew there would be short-term consequences. Nancy herself acknowledged this. We had all agreed to ride it out—because setting higher standards for our grants was best for Komen and because we wanted out of the middle of Planned Parenthood's issues and the abortion fight; we didn't want to continue spending our time and resources—even losing financial support—defending Komen because of another organization's issues. I was upset with myself for the mistakes I had made in not better anticipating how Planned Parenthood would attack. I was angry at what I believed was betrayal by my Komen teammates and our own consultants. And I was deeply disappointed that Nancy had not had the courage to stand up for Komen and what she knew was the best decision for our organization.

I remain convinced that Komen should have stood firm—at least through the weekend. Nothing would have been worse on Monday than it was Friday—and arguably, with a series of editorials set to run, including one by Robert George in the *Wall*

Street Journal, it well could have improved. From the beginning, I believed that if the issue broke into the media we could not win on that field—that's why I steadfastly pushed for a statement-only response. The media's true bias was exposed for all to see, and I now understood better than ever that the mainstream media is part of the liberal establishment and served as willing lieutenants in Planned Parenthood's army. The media chose its side right from the start.

In a *Huffington Post* article about the reversal, an anonymous Komen insider said that I was "horrified" about Komen "caving" and that I was "politically tone-deaf" for continuing to advocate that Komen stay the course.[5] I was struck by the so-called insider's comments. The words had the ring of victory to them. Why would anyone close to Komen use the word *caving* to characterize the reversal? I wondered whose side this person was really on. I also knew that this person had to be close to Komen—if not inside Komen. There were only a handful of people in the D.C. office who were privy to my conversation with Nancy and Liz, and I doubted that either Liz or Nancy would have told many others. I also found irony in now being called "politically tone-deaf," when for the past week, I was disparaged as a savvy political operative with an anti-abortion agenda doing the bidding of the Christian right.

That Friday afternoon, I was scheduled to be on a one-o'clock flight home to Atlanta. I let Liz know this when she advised me of a call with our affiliates that afternoon. Liz replied that "all leaders" would be on the call. Though I vehemently disagreed with Komen's decision to reverse course, I respected that the decision had been made and knew that my professional obligation was to join Liz and Nancy in the conference room for the call. I changed my flight.

The Apology Tour

The apology tour started on that conference call. But it didn't end there. Just before the conference call, Liz sent a staff-wide announcement. It was a total reversal of the new grants policy and focused on reinstating Planned Parenthood's eligibility.

"We want to apologize to the American public for recent decisions that cast doubt upon our commitment to our mission of saving women's lives," the statement from Nancy read. "The events of this week have been deeply unsettling for our supporters, partners and friends and all of us at Susan G. Komen. We have been distressed at the presumption that the changes made to our funding criteria were done for political reasons or to specifically penalize Planned Parenthood. They were not. . . . We will continue to fund existing grants, including those of Planned Parenthood, and preserve their eligibility to apply for future grants, while maintaining the ability of our affiliates to make funding decisions that meet the needs of their communities.

"It is our hope and we believe it is time for everyone involved to pause, slow down and reflect on how grants can most effectively and directly be administered without controversies that hurt the cause of women. We urge everyone who has participated in this conversation across the country over the last few days to help us move past this issue. We do not want our mission marred or affected by politics—anyone's politics."

My stomach turned at what I saw as a lack of honesty and sincerity in this statement. In less than seventy-two hours, we had done a complete about-face and had done so while claiming that we didn't want politics to affect what we were doing. Yet, in capitulating to Planned Parenthood and the left, Komen had done exactly what we said we would not do: politicize breast cancer. And what of the poor-quality grants that Liz and Nancy had said repeatedly did not deliver the kind of outcomes we needed for the women we served?

I found myself focused on the last two words of the statement: "anyone's politics." What did that mean? Was I the "anyone" they were referencing?

While Liz was telling our staffers that we had surrendered and it had all been a big mistake, Nancy was calling members of Congress. It seemed that Komen was trying to have it both ways—to be all things to all people. Internally at Komen, to our affiliates, and to Democrats, it was a complete reversal, with our statement clearly saying that Komen would preserve Planned Parenthood's eligibility for grants. Nancy was working the phones—apologizing to the Democrats and trying to explain to the Republicans. Word was sent to various faith-based leaders. The message for Republicans and the faith community was that Komen was only backing down for now; it would take more time to transition out of the Planned Parenthood grants. And as Komen was waving the flag of surrender, flowers from various pro-life organizations were being delivered to Nancy.

Komen had fulfilled all my worst fears. They did not have the stomach for the fight, and sadly, it was politics—not our mission—that ruled on this day. By the time I boarded the plane to Atlanta and home to Steve, I knew that I could no longer work for this organization—an organization where I had hoped to find a reprieve from politics, an organization in which I had so fully believed.

9

Leaving Komen

As the plane took off from Washington, D.C., I closed my eyes, trying to leave the week's stress and disappointment on the ground. But as soon as I was able, I powered up my iPad to check the Internet chatter on Komen's reversal. It was all cheers and celebration now that Komen had acknowledged the error of its ways and paid the ransom demand of the Planned Parenthood thugs. As I skimmed through the various Facebook posts and tweets, there it was: a tweet from Hilary Rosen.

Rosen—*our consultant*—retweeted something from Nancy Pelosi. Here's what Pelosi tweeted: "When women speak out, women win—Komen decision to continue funding Planned Parenthood is a victory for women's health."[1] A few minutes later, Rosen (@hilaryr) had tweeted herself: "Congrats to Susan G. Komen for the Cure. . . . No room for politics in fighting cancer."[2]

These were the bullies to whom we had caved. And they knew all along that we would cave.

Leaving Komen

I landed in Atlanta early that evening. I was supposed to be back in Dallas on Monday. That night, I told my husband I wasn't going; I was resigning. He already knew that would be my decision; he knew me that well. I spoke with two lawyers and my longtime friend Rob Simms throughout the weekend. One approach was to wait it out and see what, if any, move Komen would make—because, after all, I was simply doing my job. But I wanted out and didn't want this to string along. The other option was to resign. Rob was blunt as usual. "Walk away immediately." I talked to Rae Forker Evans, too.

For one of the few times in my life, I did not know what to do.

On Sunday, I sent Liz a note, letting her know that I was planning to work from home in Atlanta on Monday and that I'd head to D.C. on Tuesday to deal with various other issues. I told her I'd keep my distance from anything related to Planned Parenthood. To that point, I'd heard nothing from anyone at all—radio silence. Not even so much as a phone call from Liz.

On Monday, Nancy called. The liberal jackals had moved on from me to Nancy by now, proof that once you give in to a bully, they come back for more. She was concerned about her future and sounded truly distraught. I had underestimated the level of animosity and envy toward Nancy and Komen generally, even from some of Komen's strongest allies. Many people seemed to be reveling in the black smudge on the pink ribbon. While certain board members may have entertained the idea of ousting her, doing so would be no easy task. She was the founder of Komen and had built it into the world's top breast cancer organization, in her sister's honor. I, for one, thought it was a significant injustice to Nancy for anyone to attempt to limit her involvement in Komen.

Nancy kept asking if I was okay, but I thought that what she was really asking is what was I going to do. I made sure that I didn't say much—just that I was thinking through my options.

We finished the call. A few minutes later, she called back, saying she thought that something could be worked out. She kept apologizing and saying that I deserved it; that Steve and I deserved it—some type of financial consideration because I had been doing my job. It bothered me that she kept apologizing. I think because it only served to underscore what I felt: that she knew I had done my job and the apology was more about the fact that I was being hung out to dry. She also kept saying that we'd work out something, that she was sure the board would agree. I suggested we talk the following morning, on Tuesday.

My next call was to Mike Bowers, former attorney general of Georgia and a close friend. I was upset and wavering, uncharacteristically unsure. I *was* doing my job and now I was being made the scapegoat. A severance would at least give Steve and me some cushion. But if I took a severance, everyone would assume that I had acted improperly—that the media reports were true. I'd have money but *this* would be the story of my life. And it simply felt wrong to take a severance from a nonprofit and slink away.

Throughout the day, I talked to each of my closest friends and to my pastor. I talked to my sister. Steve and I went over our options again and again.

I called Mike again. He knew me well and sensed my angst. He finally said, "Karen, I've got to take off my lawyer hat and just be your friend. You have two choices. What is your priority? You can look at this from the perspective of the severance—which you most certainly are entitled to. Or you can think about it in terms of your reputation and being able to set the record straight. I will help you and support you in whatever you decide."

Without skipping a beat, I said, "Obviously, the latter."

He said, "That's the Karen Handel I know. And all I've got to say to you now is: It's time to cowgirl up." All I could think of was the fact that I didn't own any spurs.

But, as soon as I said it out loud, I knew I had to leave on my own terms. I had an immediate sense of calm and resolve. I knew what I wanted and needed to do for my husband, for me, and for Komen.

Setting the Record Straight

Here in Georgia, reporters were emailing, calling, tweeting, knocking on the front door. Camping out. My friend Dan, who had handled press on the campaign, knew we had to release the valve a little bit. We mapped out a plan. I would write my resignation letter, get the lawyers' sign-off, and call Nancy the next morning. We would do press that afternoon. Dan's Atlanta home would be the media base.

At 10 a.m., I called Nancy. I told her that I was resigning

immediately. She said how sorry she was that it had all come to this and said that she would talk with the board to work out a severance.

"Respectfully," I said, "I decline."

Her response was silence. I think I had caught her off guard.

Nancy spent the next ten minutes or so trying to convince me to reconsider the severance. She said that Steve and I needed to be able to take care of ourselves; that we deserved that. Again, I declined. "I'm not interested," I said. This was about self-respect. I was not going to demean myself by skulking away from a non-profit after doing nothing wrong.

I also let Nancy know that I was going to do several press interviews. I had no obligation to share this with her, but I wanted her to know out of professional courtesy and respect. Regardless of how I felt, I did my best to remain a professional. I told her I would do only a limited number of interviews—press here in Georgia and Megyn Kelly's show on Fox News. After that I would go silent. I said that I hoped she would understand that I had to say *something* to get the press to back off.

So we got ready. As soon as I finished my call with Nancy, I emailed my resignation letter. Meanwhile, Steve had set up a Facebook page and posted the letter there. I wanted to say it first rather than the press reporting it. Dan distributed the resignation letter to the media. Then Steve and I headed to Dan's.

Gathered in Dan's kitchen, the island covered with three iPads and two Macs, we worked through my talking points while trying to stop Dan's 165-pound Saint Bernard from leaving too much slobber on us. I would acknowledge my involvement. I was going to call Planned Parenthood out for what they were—bullies who had taken advantage of Komen; who were willing to destroy a breast cancer organization for their own political motives. I was going to be as positive about Komen as I could.

Press began showing up. Dan and Steve managed the reporters while I finalized what I was going to say.

First up was the Fox interview with Kelly. I was uneasy, a bit nervous, but determined. "I clearly acknowledge that I was involved in the process," I told her, "but to suggest that I had the sole authority is just absurd. The process was vetted, the policies were vetted at all of the appropriate levels in the organization." "Komen was doing its best to get to neutral ground." I specifically took direct aim at Planned Parenthood: "private nonprofit organizations have a right and a responsibility to be able to set the highest standards and criteria. Let alone the level of vicious attacks and coercion that has occurred by Planned Parenthood. It's simply outrageous. . . . The only group here that has made this issue political has been Planned Parenthood."

As soon as I finished the interview, I had a text. It was from Nancy's chief of staff. He commended me on a great interview.

Next, my cell rang. It was Nancy. She seemed to gush right through the phone about the interview—how great it was. She told me she couldn't believe how poised and professional I was, just amazing, how she was so grateful.

After everything that had taken place, after being made the scapegoat for a group decision and voluntarily walking the plank, after receiving death threats . . . after all of it, this was the lowest moment of all. Nancy seemed to be calling to breathe a sigh of relief over the fact that I hadn't stabbed Komen in the back. "Nancy," I said, "I appreciate your call. But I have to ask, do you really think so little of me that you thought I would go out and skewer Komen? I'm a professional, and I was always willing to do my job. That wasn't the problem. The problem was the lack of leadership; the lack of courage to see through what we all agreed was in Komen's best interest." It wasn't an antagonistic conversation, but I felt I had to let her know how I really felt about it all.

Several people from Komen told me that, in the moments leading up to the Kelly interview, Komen employees were gathered around TVs to watch. Afterward, more than one Komen employee asked why I had not done the press interviews all along. Liz Thompson was there and I was told that she watched the Fox interview in tears. Why she cried, I really don't know.

A week or so later, Liz left me a voice-mail message. It was the first time she'd called since I'd left Komen. "Hello, Karen," she said. "It's Liz. I just wanted to say again that you have exhibited nothing but grace and the most noble of leadership characteristics. Your television interview was masterful. As I said in my note to you, I listened humbly and had tears running down my face the entire time and then read your exchange [comments] today in the *Daily Beast*. You are an extraordinary human being, and I am sorry that this has all unfolded in the way that it did. I know that you are today acting out of the depths of the leadership characteristics you have and that you will continue down that path with an amazing life ahead. Wishing you all the best and thinking only best thoughts for you. Hope that at some point we can reconnect and just wanted again to let you know how proud I am of you and how absolutely extraordinary you are. Take care."

It seemed that Liz did not blame me. But blame wasn't really the issue. The biggest issue is that no one in Komen's leadership had the confidence or courage to stand by me when they knew I had been doing my job all along. I became a convenient scapegoat. And Komen had given in to the schoolyard bullies. There's only one way to deal with a bully: stand up and punch her in the nose. I was sad that Komen—and Nancy—had not been able or willing to do so. Don't get me wrong, I appreciated the enormous pressure they faced. But it just seemed to me that it was easier to appease Planned Parenthood than to fight back, even if that meant continuing with grants that weren't delivering what Komen really needed and were continuing to distract the organization from its real mission. I was the lunch money that Planned Parenthood demanded; the grants were the bus fare.

The Planned Bullyhood had won and would most certainly move on to its next target, identifying a new victim; seeking a new ransom.

My Bonus

The next day, reporters were still knocking on the door. We packed our bags, loaded our pups Maggie and Mia into the car, and headed to Savannah. I did my best to sweat out the stress of the past ten days with long runs through the diverse neighborhoods of Georgia's first state capital. Steve and I walked on the beaches of Tybee Island, mostly silent, just glad to have some quiet time together.

Over the next two weeks, things cooled down. The Obama campaign, the media, and lefties, they all moved on to the next target as they worked to make their case that Republicans were waging a war on women: Rush Limbaugh. For the record, he should not have said what he said about Sandra Fluke, but as the facts came forward, it was clear that his poorly chosen words launched a liberal attack that was already primed and ready to go, just waiting for the right moment. Bullies always have a next target. The usual suspects—Planned Parenthood, Media Matters, the Obama administration, the press—were doing their best to drive boycotts of Limbaugh's advertisers and pillory him as a sexist.

About two weeks later, a Google alert popped. Komen was polling. The poll, unbelievably, was testing *my* favorables versus unfavorables when lined up against people like Barbara Boxer and Nancy Pelosi. Nancy Brinker's name was listed, too. Another section of the poll was a series of positioning statements in which people were asked, "As you read this statement, does it make you more or less likely to donate to Komen?" One statement, which someone in the media dubbed "throw Karen Handel under the bus," said this: "We have made recent mistakes, which we thoroughly regret. The person at the center of the controversy, former Susan G. Komen Senior Vice President, has left the organization. We look forward to putting this behind us and fully focusing on our mission to end breast cancer."[3]

I could not believe this was happening. I was livid. So was

Steve. As I called Nancy Brinker, Steve gave me the "be calm" signal. This poll implied to the whole world that I was the root of all that had happened—it was essentially confirming all the lies that the media and blogs had reported. Nancy picked up immediately. I didn't waste time on pleasantries. I said, "I want an explanation about this poll." She said she didn't know anything about it. I suggested that she find out—right then—and call me back.

Ten minutes later she called back.

"Now, Karen, let me explain. You don't understand. You don't understand. We have to do this poll," she protested. "We have to figure out what to say!"

My response was simple: "Here's an idea: how about the truth?"

"You don't understand."

"No, Nancy," I said, "*you* don't understand. Komen needs to pull that poll."

She actually fought back, saying, "You're a public figure; we can have whatever we want in this poll."

I could not believe this. I had walked away voluntarily. I even did so without taking a cent. I did an interview defending Komen. And this was my thanks?

"Okay," I replied. "If you want to go down this road, fine. I'm a public figure. But in this instance, I was a Komen employee doing my job. There is a professional and appropriate way to handle the situation, and this is beyond inappropriate. I have a lawyer, Nancy, and he's the former attorney general of the state of Georgia. He describes himself as 'the meanest lawyer you've ever met in your life.' So you can pull the poll or you'll hear from him tomorrow morning."

The poll was pulled. Just a few days later, a new poll was released, and this one met with a harsh response from the media, ripping Komen for wasting money on a poll instead of spending it on breast cancer programs. That poll too was quickly pulled. But the fact that they were polling in the first place just to determine what to say told me all I needed to know. The Planned Bullyhood really had won, intimidating Komen to such an extent that the organization was going to do and say whatever was necessary to meet the demands of the left.

What Next?

After securing their ransom in full in just three days, Planned Parenthood and the left moved on to other targets. Ironically, what slowed the "war on women" theme was a blunder by none other than Hilary Rosen. Rosen announced on national television that Ann Romney, wife of Republican candidate Mitt Romney, hadn't worked a day in her life, this despite the fact that Mrs. Romney raised five children while suffering through breast cancer and multiple sclerosis. Komen would have done much better to ally with Ann Romney than Rosen.

It was typical Rosen. She was a Democratic propagandist, first and foremost. She had kept her status as a liberal shill during her entire time consulting for Komen. And what of her congratulatory tweet that there was no politics in fighting breast cancer? That took a backseat when it came to attacking a Republican breast cancer survivor.

And what of Komen? Since that week, the Planned Parenthood episode seems to be the reason for anything that goes wrong at Komen. Certainly, the episode has hurt the organization, and I can understand their desire to find a reason, but it's dishonest. As I said earlier, Komen was already facing financial and organizational challenges. Fund-raising had hit a wall, and we all knew that the organization could no longer afford to turn away any group of potential donors. But a scapegoat is a convenient thing, and so for now, the Planned Parenthood fiasco, as the press routinely refers to it, along with me to a certain extent, continue to serve as culprits.

Several key Komen executives have left the organization. Katrina McGhee announced her resignation just a month or so after the Planned Parenthood firestorm. I wasn't surprised. I believe that she knew that with or without the Planned Parenthood issue, some rocky times were ahead. Leslie Aun has also moved on, as have several others. The demands for Nancy's resignation have died down, and I'm glad for that. Nancy built Komen and made it what it is today—and there is far more good about the organization than bad.

In trying to increase the quality and outcomes of its grants and, in the process, move away from Planned Parenthood, Komen made an appropriate decision for the organization; for the mission. Unfortunately, in caving to the demands of Planned Parenthood and the left, Komen gave credence to the criticism that it was about politics all along. Worse, in total surrender, I fear that Komen has made itself even more vulnerable to bullies who almost always come back for more. It's my hope that people will consider Komen's tremendous contributions over the past thirty years, and instead of trying to shred the pink ribbon, work with Komen to patch it up. The one in eight women who will be diagnosed with breast cancer in their lifetime depend on it.

As for Planned Parenthood? Planned Parenthood took full advantage of Komen's weaknesses—and its kindness. Planned Parenthood and their liberal partners viciously attacked a good organization for their own political gain. Unless Planned Parenthood and its elite liberal forces are stopped, what they did to Komen is just the beginning.

Conclusion

The political aftermath of Planned Parenthood's attack on Komen was clear: the Democrats, with Planned Parenthood as their mafia-style enforcers, achieved their goal—and made their point. Women—specifically in the "war on women"—were once again front and center. The message: anyone attempting to defy the liberal guard does so at their own peril.

Komen dared to do just that in order to do what was best for the organization and its mission and, in the process, forced a confrontation with the left and its abortion zealots. For this sin, Planned Parenthood unleashed a swift and devastating assault, securing the breast cancer organization's surrender in just seventy-two hours. With the expert precision and mass scale of its offensive, Planned Parenthood delivered the time-honored message of all bullies: do what we say or we will make you pay. Planned Parenthood won the same way bullies always win— pummeling the victim from all sides and counting on no one to have the courage to stand up and face them down. And just as the abuser blames the abused, saying "she had it coming," Planned Parenthood, the Democratic establishment, and even the media, put the blame on Komen with their hypocritical exclamations that implied "Planned Parenthood had no choice"; "Komen had it coming."

———

By mid-April 2011, polls had Democrats beating Republicans on the congressional level by 10 points—a 51 percent to 41 percent margin. While women had actually voted in majorities for Republicans in 2010, the so-called war on women—a trumped-up conflict supposedly led by conservatives declared by liberals like Barack Obama, Cecile Richards, and Hilary Rosen—had put women squarely back into the Democratic column. As Democratic pollsters Stan Greenberg and Page Gardner wrote, "In the Republican-held districts where we have data from last year, Democrats picked up a net 10 points among women since December and now lead by 4 points. Among unmarried women, Democrats lead by 20 points in Republican held districts."[1] The Planned Parenthood bullying strategy and its metamorphosis into a women's health organization rather than an abortion provider was having the desired effect. Planned Parenthood's $1.4 million ad campaign against the Romney launch in June also seemed to be making an impact. A poll conducted by Politico and the Hart Institute of those women who remembered seeing the ad showed that Romney's overall image was hurt among women since the ad began airing. Politico and the Hart Institute concede that it's possible that those who remembered the ads were also already inclined to be supportive of the ad's themes. Nevertheless, the ads seemed to be making a mark.[2]

The polling heading into November will no doubt shift back

and forth over the course of the political campaign cycle. It remains unclear right now where the votes of women will go.

But what is clear is this: Planned Parenthood is a powerful and effective combat weapon for the left, willing to put its own political agenda—abortion and its government funding—ahead of women. Planned Parenthood is waging a *real* war on women, and it's waging that war on multiple fronts.

In attacking Komen, Planned Parenthood purposely tried to destroy a good organization doing great work on behalf of women. Planned Parenthood dismissed the decades-long partnership with Komen with cruelty and callousness and no appreciation for the millions that Komen had granted to it over the years. Komen extended every professional courtesy to the organization it thought was a friend, but that didn't stop Planned Parenthood from stabbing its friend in the back. Planned Parenthood willingly made Komen collateral damage, caring nothing for the women that Komen supports through its grant dollars—dollars that would have been invested elsewhere to help even more women.

Planned Parenthood executed a flawless campaign against Komen, so much so that it begs the question whether there was inside help. Indeed, the coincidences are so prevalent that it seems nearly impossible that all of them were mere happenstance. Consider: Komen made its decision in early December and Komen president Liz Thompson spoke with Planned Parenthood CEO Cecile Richard in mid-December. Cecile already knew about the decision. In November, Komen hired Hilary Rosen, noted Democratic talking head and a principal in the

PR firm SKDKnickerbocker. SKDKnickerbocker counts among its principals Anita Dunn, former Obama White House communications director, and Emily Lenzner, whom Hilary called the firm's Planned Parenthood expert. SKDKnickerbocker lays claim to having delivered Obama's first White House win on its website, touting its extensive role. Hilary Rosen and Cecile Richards are frequent visitors to the White House. Cecile Richards is an Obama confidante, serving as key counsel on women's health issues. Komen's other consultant, Ogilvy's Brandon Daly, is a former colleague of Planned Parenthood CEO Cecile Richards. They worked together for Nancy Pelosi. Hilary Rosen and Emily Lenzner just happened to be in the Komen offices meeting with Komen Communications vice president Leslie Aun on the very day that Associated Press called about the issue. That same day, DNC Chairman Debbie Wasserman Schultz had a prescheduled call with Nancy Brinker. The Associated Press story came out late afternoon on January 31, but *Huffington Post* already had the article up. Several blog posts and tweets went out the day *before* the Associated Press story hit. Senator Patty Murray (D-WA) had a statement finalized and ready to go within a very short time after story broke. The Associated Press story coincided with the premiere of the *Pink Ribbons, Inc.* documentary that is critical of Komen and its marketing practices. Planned Parenthood had fundraising appeals in in-boxes within an hour. Other Democratic organizations and online petition organizations were on the ready, too. Congressman Mike Honda (D-CA) had his "dear colleague" letter distributed to his House colleagues the very next day, while on the Senate side, a similar letter had secured the signatures of more than twenty senators in equally record time. Nancy Brinker was on the air saying that politics had not played a role in the decision, and almost simultaneously, a story in the *Atlantic* magazine broke that quoted Komen sources contradicting her. Meanwhile, the Obama administration was pushing the contraception mandate and preparing to go all-in with its "Republican war on women" theme.

There are other coincidences in this extraordinary chain of events, but I'll stop here and let you decide. Were all of these occurrences just a matter of chance? Or was it something more? For me, there is only one logical answer. Planned Parenthood and their Democratic associates at the DNC and the White House saw a political opportunity in Komen's ill-timed decision and seized the moment. They orchestrated a premeditated assault to spread Planned Parenthood's propaganda that it is a general women's health-care organization rather than the country's leading abortion provider and to advance the "Republican war on women" refrain, which is now a central Obama campaign theme. Today, the Obama campaign is running TV ads paying specific and high homage to Planned Parenthood and assailing Mitt Romney for his position that the abortion provider should not receive federal funding.[3]

Planned Parenthood says it's the champion for women. But their public persona hides a harsh and shocking reality: Planned Parenthood is more assailant than advocate.

Not content with a war on living women, Planned Parenthood is now waging war against unborn girls.

In May 2012, Lila Rose's Live Action released two videos

showing Planned Parenthood employees providing support and aid to women who wanted to abort their female babies—women who wanted late-term sex-selective abortions. "This was a multistate, national investigation demonstrating that this is a widespread problem across our country," said Live Action president Lila Rose. "First of all, the statistics and studies indicate that we are adding to the growing problem across the world of sex-selective targeting of unborn girls for abortion. We are going to be demonstrating . . . that the abortion industry in the United States is aiding and abetting this horrific problem." A full 77 percent of Americans want to ban sex-selective abortions.[4]

Planned Parenthood protested, saying the tapes were a hoax—the same excuse they've given each time a sordid detail is uncovered about them. "Planned Parenthood does not offer sex determination services; our ultrasound services are limited to medical purposes," said Planned Parenthood education top executive Leslie Kantor and senior medical advisor Carolyn Westhoff. "Gender bias is contrary to everything our organization works for daily in communities across the country. Planned Parenthood opposes racism and sexism in all forms, and we work to advance equity and human rights in the delivery of health care."[5]

More spin and evasiveness. Planned Parenthood's spokeswoman went on to explain that its job was to make available "high quality, confidential, nonjudgmental care to all who come."[6] How could any organization that proclaimed itself the champions of women not condemn outright and unequivocally the appalling practice of sex-selective abortions?

Not only that—when Republican congressmen tried to pass

a bill banning sex-selective abortion, Planned Parenthood said "it strongly opposes legislation in the House that would impose harmful restrictions on women's health care and interfere with the doctor/patient relationship. . . . The bill also fails to address the real causes of inequality and health disparities and in fact takes aim at the very communities it claims to help. Racism and gender discrimination are serious issues, yet this bill would cast suspicion on doctors that serve communities facing the greatest health disparities, many of which are minority communities." In other words, Planned Parenthood, which just spent months claiming to be fighting *for* women, is now *against* protecting unborn girls from gendercide. Their claims of racism and sexism as a justification are a thin excuse for such despicable acts.[7]

The intimacy between Planned Parenthood and the Obama administration was evident when the president found himself defending sex-selective abortion as part of a woman's right to choose . . . to kill future women. White House deputy press secretary Jamie Smith told Jake Tapper of ABC News, "The administration opposes gender discrimination in all forms"— well, all forms except killing girls based on gender—"but the end result of this legislation would be to subject doctors to criminal prosecution if they fail to determine the motivations behind a very personal and private decision. The government should not intrude in medical decisions or private family matters in this way."[8]

This latest Planned Parenthood revelation has not only fueled disgust, it has provided new steam to legislatures around the country seeking to cut off state funding to the organization. In North Carolina, House legislators passed a budget that would prohibit funding to providers of "family planning" and "pregnancy prevention"—in other words, Planned Parenthood, since that's the only organization in North Carolina that fits this definition. North Carolina had tried to enact this prohibition the year before, but Planned Parenthood sued and was able to find a judge to overturn the funding ban. Planned Parenthood then raked in about $343,000 in taxpayer cash. North Carolina Governor Bev Perdue (D-NC) vetoed the bill, but the state legislature voted to override her veto. Ironically, the new executive director for one of Komen's North Carolina affiliates once headed up a Planned Parenthood chapter. She said in a recent interview that her goal with Komen is to "reduce politics."[9]

North Carolina isn't alone in moving to bar Planned Parenthood from receiving state funding. Thirteen other states have stopped funding Planned Parenthood.[10]

Months later, I can only wonder how Komen feels about its decision to cave. *This* is the organization it surrendered to—an organization that put politics and money above the fight against breast cancer; an organization that refuses to condemn the practice of sex-selective abortions; an organization so controversial, so divisive, that more than a dozen states across the country are moving to defund it; an organization whose grants are crappy, as Liz called them, and that fails to achieve real results that will advance the fight against breast cancer. I suspect that it's only a matter of time before Komen once again finds itself at this same crossroads about Planned Parenthood. Only time will tell what path Komen will take; whether the next time, Komen will have the stomach for a fight.

The broader question, though, is whether the bully tactics of the left will secure an unconditional victory in the end. The campaign started with Komen, but it certainly didn't end with Komen. And it won't end until we, as Americans, stand up to the perverse tactics of thugs like Planned Parenthood—and the politicians they pay for to do their dirty work.

Planned Bullyhood's Impact

With its network of political action committees and a willing army of devoted, vocal supporters, Planned Parenthood has honed its political combat tactics and is poised to shape elections today and well into the future. With Komen, they achieved something they never had before: the public near destruction of a widely trusted and passionately supported organization dedicated to nonpolitical goals. This has broad ramifications. Planned Parenthood has opened the door to a shakedown of American politics by liberal interest groups, employing mafia-style tactics to hold hostage sponsors and advertisers and even other nonprofits that dare to defy their agenda or support those who do.

Other liberal groups have figured out that the Planned Parenthood strategy works—and they have been emboldened to replicate the tactic. Virtually every organization on the left now knows that it's possible to bully private organizations into submission and silence with the help of government allies and media friends.

Just a few weeks after Komen's cave-in, Rush Limbaugh went on the air to discuss Sandra Fluke, a radical feminist activist who had just been called by Democrats to testify before Congress on the contraception issue. Fluke was portrayed by the media as your average college student. It turned out that Fluke was actually thirty and had specifically enrolled at Georgetown Law School so that she could challenge the fact that the religious school didn't cover her contraceptive care. This, of course, was just a few short weeks after the Obama administration had announced its contraception mandate, trampling religious freedom.

Rush Limbaugh proceeded to say:

> What does it say about the college co-ed Susan [*sic*] Fluke, who goes before a congressional committee and essentially says that she must be paid to have sex, what does that make her? It makes her a slut, right? It makes her a prostitute. She wants to be paid to have sex. She's having so much sex she can't afford the contraception. She wants you and me and the taxpayers to pay her to have sex. . . . Okay, so she's not a slut. She's "round heeled." I take it back.

It was inflammatory, completely inappropriate language. To his credit, Limbaugh apologized—as he should have. To their discredit, Republican leaders were largely silent. Their silence echoed the quiet of my fellow Republicans during the Georgia governor's race when Georgia Right to Life made its heinous "barren" and "desperate" comments about Steve and me and others like us who pursued fertility treatments. In leadership, it's not enough to call out the other side when something inappropriate is said or done. We have to be willing to hold our own accountable as well.

Limbaugh's apology came too late, and the muted response from Republicans was an unforced error that allowed the left to run with the issue. Planned Parenthood and its friends pounced on the remarks as an opportunity to lead a campaign against Limbaugh and his advertisers. Barack Obama, sensing a political opportunity, personally called Sandra Fluke, saying that she shouldn't be attacked because she was a private citizen. (I'm still waiting for my call from President Obama.) Nancy Pelosi attacked Limbaugh. So did seventy-five Democrats who signed a letter condemning Limbaugh—after he had already apologized.

Fluke refused to accept the apology and began her media tour. Ironically, the same public relations firm that was supposed to help Komen effectively manage the left and Planned Parenthood was managing Fluke's PR: Hilary Rosen's SKDKnickerbocker. Fluke's talking points were even richer in irony. She would say that she expected criticism but not personal attacks. I wonder how Planned Parenthood and the "Leftinistas" reconciled their personal attacks on me as they condemned others during the Fluke incident? Where was Hilary Rosen on the Sunday morning political shows denouncing the personal attacks against me?

Soon Obama's minions in the nonprofit world were leading an effort to boycott Limbaugh's show at the local level. MoveOn.org, Media Matters, Think Progress, Daily Kos—all the same groups that rallied to Planned Parenthood's side against Komen—targeted advertisers on Limbaugh's show, telling the companies that they would essentially destroy their businesses if the ads were not pulled.

Limbaugh stood up to them and refused to be bullied. He's still on the air. But the campaign against Limbaugh continues.

These tactics have now become a mainstay of the left with the mainstream media as their allies.

Next came the campaigns against conservative organizations like the American Legislative Exchange Council (ALEC) for its support of voter photo ID laws and "stand your ground" laws. Democratic legislators—and their allies like the Van Jones–led Color of Change organization—decided to target ALEC, saying these laws were racist.

Ironically, my work on Georgia's voter photo ID law was one of the liberal rallying cries against me during Planned Parenthood's attack on Komen. Requiring voters to show a photo ID is a commonsense voter integrity program. Those bringing race into the debate are off base. In Georgia, African American voter turnout was up 42 percent from 2004 to 2008 and white turnout increased 8 percent during this period.[11] Not a single individual in Georgia has been denied the right to vote because of this requirement.

The outcry over ALEC and these legislative proposals was ridiculous, just as it was ridiculous to suggest that Komen was a tool of right-wing crazies because Komen wanted to invest the dollars that were going to substandard Planned Parenthood grants elsewhere in order to better serve more women.

Soon, Color of Change, with help from friends at outlets like *Huffington Post*, joined the gang of bullies targeting companies that supported ALEC. Hilary Rosen was even extolling the evils of voter photo ID. And the campaign worked. To date, more than twenty prominent corporations, including Wal-Mart, Coca-Cola, Pepsi, Kraft, John Deere, HP, CVS Caremark, and Best Buy have disassociated from ALEC. These companies pulled their support despite the fact that ALEC, like Komen, had caved quickly. ALEC announced that it would no longer involve itself in issues such as voter ID legislation and "stand your ground" laws and, instead, retreated to the safer ground of economic policy. Yet, the left has not relented. But as I have said before, simply giving in to a bully is rarely enough. A bully must exact a price.

Indeed, the media in many cases have assumed the roles of advocates instead of journalists. In covering the Komen/Planned Parenthood story, Andrea Mitchell designated herself as the standard bearer for "expressing the anger of the people" in her interview with Nancy Brinker. I have no doubt that Mitchell was personally angry. But that's not really the point. The point is that Mitchell allowed her personal feelings and affinity for Planned Parenthood to supplant even the feeblest attempt to convey the facts and present an objective report.

I first experienced the liberal media bias in my days with Marilyn Quayle, when Vice President Dan Quayle was their target. There are so many other examples—from the media's disgraceful treatment of Sarah Palin to its portrayal of the Tea Party. And, more than two months after the Live Action tapes were released, the three network news programs had still not covered the Planned Parenthood sex-selection abortion issue. Yet the Komen/Planned Parenthood issue enjoyed extensive coverage.[12]

Sadly and disturbingly, the line between journalism and activism has all but been erased.

The truth seems not to matter much these days. What matters most is the activism of the radical left and their allies in government and the media to push the liberal causes and candidates.

You don't have to take my word for how effective these bully tactics have been. The liberals already know. In early June, a political fund-raising piece landed in the mailboxes of Georgians. The headline screamed "Online Activism Works." The three photos plastered just under this headline? Pictures of Limbaugh, a bottle of Coca-Cola, and me.

The fix is in. And it was patented by Planned Parenthood.

What We Can Do

This battle has just begun. In order for it to end in victory for the First Amendment, for freedom of association, for the freedom to choose whom and what to fund, we—you and I—must find the courage to stand up to groups like Planned Parenthood. To be sure, bullying exists on the right as well as the left, and I, for one, will not condone it on either side. But the bullying from the left is much more dangerous, because it comes with the seal of approval from government and the media.

The bad guys have to be stopped.

One of the first steps in stopping them is ending government funding to Planned Parenthood.

It should concern all of us that an overtly political interest group like Planned Parenthood receives nearly $500 million a year—that's nearly $1.5 million each and every day—in government funding. It should shock us all that Planned Parenthood played an influential role in shaping Obamacare, a health reform law that would add millions in government funding to Planned Parenthood's revenue line and covertly establishes coverage for elective abortion services by insurance plans in the state health exchanges along with a required abortion surcharge.

Planned Parenthood's funding is legally funneled to its many political arms to be doled out to candidates who will be Planned Parenthood champions for yet more government funding. Our tax dollars enable Planned Parenthood to free up other dollars that are then used for blatantly partisan political campaigning. Already in the 2012 election cycle, Planned Parenthood has launched a $1.4 million TV ad campaign and its website (www .womenarewatching.org) regularly regurgitates the latest DNC and Obama message points. Meanwhile, Planned Parenthood CEO Cecile Richards is one of Obama's top surrogates, traveling the country to headline rallies that so aggressively promote President Obama and bash presumptive GOP nominee Mitt Romney, they should qualify as official campaign events. It should concern us all that *any* nonprofit can use its charitable status as a shield for patently partisan politics, attacking candidates of one political party almost exclusively.

A corrupt triangle has been empowered: government money flows to Planned Parenthood; Planned Parenthood money is then used to attack its opponents and elect its friends; those friends funnel more taxpayer money to Planned Parenthood. Without their permission, the American taxpayers—that's you and me—have been turned into subsidizers not only of abortion but also of political propagandizing. This must end.

Organizations like Komen also have to prepare their armor. The left has realized that, while it can bring pressure to bear on the likes of Rush Limbaugh, Limbaugh won't back down. Instead the left has discovered the soft underbelly of politics: organizations and corporate enterprises so fearful of boycotts, loss of donations, and damage to their brand that they will capitulate and pay the ransom, rather than stand and fight—even when they are on just ground.

Groups like Komen need to toughen up in the face of criticism. Certainly, negative press, emails, and blog postings are tough to take and even detrimental to an organization, but the real harm comes when the good guys—or gals, in this case—acquiesce to the demands of the bullies. Caving in emboldens the bullies, but when companies stand up to them, those companies almost always win. When Komen was holding its ground against Planned Parenthood—for all of seventy-two hours—our donations skyrocketed. Today it's been widely reported that Komen's contributions are down. As is typical of the biased media, it's always reported as a residual decline from still angry pro–Planned Parenthood donors. I suppose that's some of it, but Komen gave in to Planned Parenthood, so why haven't Planned Parenthood and its cronies on the left called off the dogs? It seems just as likely to me—if not more so—that those on the right who were Komen supporters, willing to give it the benefit of the doubt about Planned Parenthood, walked away when Komen didn't have the courage to stand up for its own mission.

The American people understand the threat posed by Planned Parenthood and its friends. Americans have a long history of confronting bullies—and winning. They won't tolerate these tactics for long. Komen and organizations like them should put a little trust and faith in the innate common sense of the American people. I firmly believe that, if Komen had stayed the course and stared down the bullies at Planned Parenthood, the American people would have rallied to Komen's aid. Unfortunately, Komen didn't give them that chance.

At Komen, our biggest mistake was in being so apolitical that we failed to recognize that our enemies weren't. We didn't know what was coming, because we were focused on the mission of fighting breast cancer; we were focused on the women we served. They were not. To fight a battle against those who would destroy you, you first have to acknowledge that you're in a fight.

And we—the American people—are in a fight. It's a fight we can win. But it won't be easy.

It's not just the pro-life issue or women's health that's at stake. It's the right of organizations to make decisions they deem necessary and appropriate without fear of threats and boycotts. It's the health of the political discourse in our country. It's the ability of those with differing political viewpoints to have an impact on the issues that matter to them without fear of reprisal and destruction—reprisal too often based on lies. Planned Parenthood is a symptom of a greater ill, and they're the tip of the spear in the left's real assault on women's health—a casualty they are willing to sacrifice in favor of political gamesmanship.

I never thought of myself as a soldier in the culture wars. My entire political life was focused more on balancing budgets, cutting taxes, streamlining processes, implementing commonsense voter laws, and being a champion for ethics. What I have come to realize from my Komen experience is this: the moment we step into the political arena, we become targets because of our beliefs—whether or not those beliefs are the issue at hand.

Planned Parenthood brought Komen to its knees, counting on no one having the guts to stand up to them. Well, what Planned Parenthood didn't count on is me. As I said before, lack of guts has never been my issue. And thanks to Planned Parenthood, I am now a new soldier—an accidental soldier, perhaps, but one who is going to stand up to them and expose them for what they really are.

The only way to stop those who politicize the apolitical, hold hostage those who dare to disagree, and bully their way to taxpayer money is to fight back.

The question is this: are we ready to fight back against these bullies? I am.

Acknowledgments

I thank God for His hand in my life and the blessings He has given me—even if sometimes they don't seem like blessings.

So many people have guided, supported, and loved me through my life. This is a simple yet heartfelt thank you to a few.

Dad, time has a way of healing and I know now that you are one of the strongest men I know. Jennifer, my wonderful sister, you teach me about real strength and faith. To Gus for being a great brother. To the GOBs, you know who you are and what you mean to me. Ally and William, you are the daughter and son we hoped to have and make us so proud every day. Rae, MQ, and Neal, you gave me a chance when most others would not; I will always be grateful and do my very best to make you glad you took a chance on me. Mike and Bette Rose, for your friendship and counsel all these years, and to you Bette Rose, the one and only "Hug Lady," for making so many people smile. To my dear friends Anne, Carol, MJ, Kathleen, and Marshall, your friendship enriches my life. Frank and Philis—I could not have done this without you. Special thanks to Ben Shapiro, who was instrumental in helping me put this story into words. Your rare wit and keen political insights make you a leading voice on today's politics and policy. Pastor Benny, you have strengthened my faith and helped me find the courage to "step out big." To Steve, you put the love and laughter in each of my days—and put up with our crazy life; I can't imagine my life without you in it. To Susan G. Komen for the Cure, an organization that has done so much for so many. And to life and irony: bring it on!

Notes

Introduction

1. *Morning Joe* (MSNBC), April 6, 2012.

2. "Andrea Mitchell interviews Susan G. Komen's Nancy Brinker," MSNBC.com, February 2, 2012, http://firstread.msnbc.msn.com/ _news/2012/02/02/10303379-andrea-mitchell-interviews-susan -g-komens-nancy-brinker?lite.

Chapter 1: Trojan Horse? Pro-Life Hero? I'm Just Karen

1. http://www.atlantada.org/latestnews/pressreleases/111403c.htm.

2. http://blogs.ajc.com/political-insider-jim-galloway/2009/05/01/ nathan-deal-promises-to-tie-his-own-shoes-announces-for -governor/.

3. http://www.gpb.org/news/2010/05/21/ethics-panel-subpoenas -oxendine-donors.

4. http://blogs.ajc.com/political-insider-jim-galloway/2010/04/29/ parents-church-and-judge-told-future-gop-candidate-for -governor-leave-the-girl-alone/.

5. http://savannahnow.com/news/2009-12-13/ethics-case-stalks -johnson-run.

6. http://savannahnow.com/news/2010–05–26/eric-johnson-ethics
-fix#.T8TwHO1uGlI.

7. http://oce.house.gov/disclosures/Review_No_09–1022_Referral_
to_Standards.pdf.

8. http://www.ajc.com/news/georgia-politics-elections/u-s-house
-panel-416361.html.

9. http://blogs.ajc.com/political-insider-jim-galloway/2010/03/22/
health-care-aftermath-nathan-deal-resigns-forces-gather-for
-counteroffensive/.

10. http://www.businessweek.com/ap/financialnews/D9I9LN2G0
.htm.

11. http://www.ajc.com/news/georgia-politics-elections/campaign
-paid-135k-to-626245.html; http://www.rollcall.com/issues/56_
39/-50822–1.html; http://www.atlantaunfiltered.com/2010/11/02/
deal-refunds-130k-in-excess-donations-cited-in-ethics-complaint/.

12. http://georgialife.wordpress.com/2010/06/03/grtl-pac-issues
-endorsement-for-governor/.

13. http://blogs.ajc.com/political-insider-jim-galloway/2010/06/03/
georgia-right-to-life-picks-a-fight-with-karen-handel/.

14. http://blogs.ajc.com/political-insider-jim-galloway/2010/06/10/
state-gop-chair-sue-everhart-has-karen-handels-back-on-pro-life
-issue/.

15. http://blogs.ajc.com/georgia_elections_news/2010/07/12/
palin-handel-ready-to-serve-as-governor/.

16. http://abcnews.go.com/Politics/sarah-palin-stumps-karen
-handel-georgia-primary-runoff/story?id=11359364&page=2#
.T8T6aO1uGlI.

17. http://www.atlantaunfiltered.com/2010/11/02/deal-refunds
-130k-in-excess-donations-cited-in-ethics-complaint/.

18. http://www.politico.com/news/stories/0810/40701.html.

Chapter 2: From the Frying Pan

1. http://thinkprogress.org/politics/2012/02/06/419680/ari-fleischer
-admits-he-personally-advised-komen-ceo-on-planned-parent
hood/.

2. Steven Ertelt, "Planned Parenthood: 51% of Its Clinic Income Comes
From Abortions," January 5, 2012, http://www.lifenews.com/2012/
01/05/planned-parenthood-51-of-its-income-comes-from
-abortions/.

3. Planned Parenthood's 2009–2010 Annual Report, http://issuu.com/
actionfund/docs/ppfa_financials_2010_122711_web_vf?mode=win
dow&viewMode=doublePage.

4. Steven Ertelt, "Planned Parenthood: 51% of Its Clinic Income Comes
From Abortions."

5. Steven Ertelt, "New Planned Parenthood Report: Record Abortions
Done in 2009," LifeNews.com, February 23, 2011, http://www
.lifenews.com/2011/02/23/new-planned-parenthood-report-record
-abortions-done-in-2009/.

6. Ezra Klein, "Repost: What Planned Parenthood actually does,
in one chart," WashingtonPost.com, February 2, 2012, http://
www.washingtonpost.com/blogs/ezra-klein/post/what-planned
-parenthood-actually-does/2011/04/06/AFhBPa2C_blog.html.

7. http://www.plannedparenthood.org/health-topics/womens
-health/breast-cancer-screenings-21189.htm.

8. "Annual Mammograms Now Recommended for Women Beginning at Age 40," American Congress of Obstetricians and Gynecologists, July 20, 2011, http://www.acog.org/About_ACOG/
News_Room/News_Releases/2011/Annual_Mammograms_
Now_Recommended_for_Women_Beginning_at_Age_40.

Chapter 3: The Gathering Storm

1. Devin Dwyer, "Undercover Video Enflames Debate Over Planned Parenthood," ABCNews.com, February 1, 2011, http://abcnews.go.com/Politics/undercover-video-enflames-debate-planned-parenthood/story?id=12814866#.T6sHeWBsg1c.

2. http://articles.latimes.com/2012/feb/03/health/la-he-komen-planned-parenthood-tictoc-20120204/2.

3. John McCormack, "After Lying About Providing Mammograms, Planned Parenthood Outraged That Breast Cancer Charity Cuts Off Grants," WeeklyStandard.com, February 2, 2012, http://www.weeklystandard.com/blogs/after-lying-about-providing-mammograms-planned-parenthood-outraged-breast-cancer-charity-cuts-grants_620875.html.

4. Josh Braham, "Pro-Lifers: Don't Support American Cancer Society Relay for Life," LifeNews.com, April 1, 2011, http://www.lifenews.com/2011/04/01/pro-lifers-dont-support-american-cancer-society-relay-for-life/.

5. http://www.nbcdfw.com/news/health/Ohio-Bishop-Bars-Support-for-Komen-125459623.html.

6. Liz Lefebvre, "Ohio bishop discourages support for Komen Foundation," August 5, 2011, http://www.uscatholic.org/blog/2011/08/ohio-bishop-discourages-support-komen-foundation.

7. "Komen Response to Toledo Bishop's Statement," July 15, 2011, KomenNEOhio.org, http://www.komenneohio.org/about-us/news/affiliate-news/komen-response-to-toledo.html.

8. "Komen for the Cure," Catholic Conference of Ohio, July 20, 2011.

9 . http://www.usatoday.com/news/health/medical/health/medical/cancer/story/2011/07/Komens-pink-ribbons-raise-green-and-questions/49472438/1.

10. http://www.onf-nfb.gc.ca/eng/press-room/index.php?id=20588.

11. Susan Tyrrell, "Sales of New Bible Help Planned Parenthood–Funding Komen," LifeNews.com, December 12, 2011, http://www.lifenews.com/2011/12/12/sales-of-new-bible-help-planned-parenthood-funding-komen/.

12. Bob Smietana, "Pink Bibles pulled after benefits tied to Planned Parenthood," *Tennesseean*, December 16, 2011, http://www.usatoday.com/news/religion/story/2011–12–15/pink-bibles-breast-cancer/51963758/1.

Chapter 4: Planned Infiltration

1. Amanda Terkel, "Susan G. Komen Head Nancy Brinker Defended PPFA In Memoir: We Can't 'Turn Our Backs On These Women,' " HuffingtonPost.com, February 7, 2012, http://www.huffingtonpost.com/2012/02/07/susan-komen-nancy-brinker-memoir-ppfa-women_n_1258761.html.

2. Rahel Musleah, "Profile: Nancy G. Brinker," *Hadassah*, December 2010/January 2011, http://www.hadassahmagazine.org/site/apps/nlnet/content.aspx?c=twI6LmN7IzF&b=5698175&ct=8965869.

3. Erin Gloria Ryan, "Nancy Brinker's Lavish Spending, Off-Putting Brittleness Puts Komen's Future In Jeopardy," Jezebel.com, February 13, 2012, http://jezebel.com/5884674/nancy-brinkers-lavish-spending-off+putting-brittleness-puts-komens-future-in-jeopardy.

4. http://www.aul.org/aul-special-report-the-case-for-investigating-planned-parenthood/.

5. http://www.awesomecapital.com/1/post/2010/9/irs-probes-sf-planned-parenthood.html.

6. http://www.lifenews.com/2011/11/03/planned-parenthood-accused-of-massive-medicaid-fraud-in-texas/.

7. http://www.kansascity.com/2011/11/09/3256411/kansas-judge-dismisses-felony.html.

8. Charlie Spiering, "Rosen hired for Wasserman-Schultz media consulting," WashingtonExaminer.com, April 12, 2012, http://campaign2012.washingtonexaminer.com/blogs/beltway-confidential/rosen-hired-wasserman-schultz-media-consulting/477051.

9. http://www.nationalreview.com/campaign-spot/295838/hilary-rosen-frequent-white-house-visitor.

Chapter 6: Once a Bully, Always a Bully

1. http://www.plannedparenthood.org/about-us/who-we-are/vision-4837.htm.

2. http://www.thenation.com/article/166670/genius-cecile-richards.

3. http://www.politico.com/blogs/bensmith/0708/Planned_Parenthood_endorses_Obama.html.

4. Planned Parenthood Annual Report for year ended June 30, 2010, http://issuu.com/actionfund/docs/ppfa_financials_2010_122711_web_vf?mode=window&viewMode=doublePage.

5. http://www.plannedparenthood.org/files/PPFA/PP_Services.pdf.

6. http://www.healthexchange.ca.gov/StakeHolders/Documents/PlannedParenthoodAffiliatesofCA-LettertotheExchangeonEER.pdf.

7. http://www.huffingtonpost.com/2012/04/02/obamacare-abortion-surcharge_n_1397564.html and http://www.catholic.org/national/national_story.php?id=45192.

8. Times Wire Services, "BRIEFING: AT&T Chief Tells Stockholders It's Planned Parenthood's Fault," *Los Angeles Times,* April 18, 1990.

9. Jill Stanek, "When Planned Parenthood tried to bully a corporate donor . . . and lost," JillStanek.com, February 7, 2012, http://www.jillstanek.com/2012/02/when-planned-parenthood-tried-to-bully-acorporate-donor-and-lost/.

10. Times Wire Services, "BRIEFING: AT&T Chief Tells Stockholders It's Planned Parenthood's Fault."

11. "AT&T Cuts Off Planned Parenthood," *Seattle Times,* April 3, 1990.

12. Stanek, "When Planned Parenthood tried to bully a corporate donor . . . and lost."

13. http://www.lifenews.com/2012/06/18/bob-evans-removed-from -planned-parenthood-donor-boycott-list/.

14. Liz Klimas, "New Planned Parenthood Condoms Use Special Codes To Show Where Users Had 'Safe Sex,' " TheBlaze.com, February 27, 2012, http://www.theblaze.com/stories/new-planned -parenthood-condoms-use-special-codes-to-show-where-users -had-safe-sex/.

15. "38.4% of Planned Parenthood's 2009 'Health Center Income' is from Abortion," LiveAction.org, April 8, 2011, http://liveaction .org/blog/38–4-of-pp-health-center-income-is-from-abortions/.

16. Steven Ertelt, "Planned Parenthood Purchases New $35M National HQ in NYC," LifeNews.com, January 25, 2012, http://www.lifenews .com/2012/01/25/planned-parenthood-purchases-new-35m -national-hq-in-nyc/.

17. Jacqueline M., "A Win for Women's Health in Pennsylvania," WomenAreWatching.org, April 27, 2012, http://www.womenare watching.org/article/a-win-for-womens-health-in-pennsylvania.

18. "Planned Parenthood Spends Big in PA Special Election," Politico .com, April 17, 2012, http://www.politico.com/blogs/burns-haber man/2012/04/planned-parenthood-spends-big-in-pennsylvania -special-120814.html.

19. Lauren Peterson, "Why Cecile Richards has President Obama's back," BarackObama.com, May 17, 2012, http://www.barack obama.com/news/entry/why-cecile-richards-has-president -obamas-back.

20. http://www.foxnews.com/politics/2012/05/30/planned-parent hood-targets-romney-with-new-swing-state-ad-buy/.

21. http://www.barackobama.com/news/entry/why-cecile-richards -has-president-obamas-back.

22. Jill Stanek, "Planned Parenthood CEO a Top White House Mandate Advisor," LifeNews.com, February 14, 2012, http://www.lifenews .com/2012/02/14/planned-parenthood-ceo-a-top-white-house -mandate-advisor/.

23. http://www.sfexaminer.com/blogs/beltway-confidential/2011/04/ planned-parenthood-spent-more-1-million-electing-democrats -last-c.

24. http://www.opensecrets.org/usearch/index.php?q=Planned+Parent hood&searchButt_clean.x=37&searchButt_clean.y=22& searchButt_clean=Submit&cx=010677907462955562473%3Anlld kv0jvam&cof=FORID%3A11.

25. http://www.skdknick.com/work/far-reaching-role-in-election/.

26. http://www.plannedparenthood.org/about-us/newsroom/press -releases/planned-parenthood-names-key-white-house-aide-dana -singiser-vice-president-public-policy-govern-38190.htm.

27. "Political and Organizing Director," May 2010, http://www.gross mansolutions.com/PPFA.pdf.

28. Sam Stein, "President Obama Leads War On Women With Economic Policies, Mitt Romney's Campaign Says," Huffington Post.com, April 10, 2012, http://www.huffingtonpost.com/2012/ 04/10/obama-war-on-women-romney_n_1416249.html.

29. Whitney Evans, "Mitt Romney widens lead over Barack Obama in new poll," DeseretNews.com, December 29, 2011, http://www .deseretnews.com/article/700210964/Mitt-Romney-widens-lead -over-Barack-Obama-in-new-poll.html.

30. Laura Bassett, "On Roe v. Wade Anniversary, Obama Vows To Protect Women's Choice," HuffingtonPost.com, January 22, 2012, http://www.huffingtonpost.com/2012/01/22/roe-v-wade _n_1222166.html.

Chapter 7: Taken Hostage

1. Katherine Clarke, "Planned Parenthood buys its NY HQ for $34.8M," TheRealDeal.com, January 24, 2012, http://therealdeal .com/blog/2012/01/24/planned-parenthood-buys-its-ny-hq-for -38-4m/.

2. Steven Ertelt, "Planned Parenthood Purchases New $35M National HQ in NYC," LifeNews.com, January 25, 2012, http://www .lifenews.com/2012/01/25/planned-parenthood-purchases-new -35m-national-hq-in-nyc/.

3. Planned Parenthood Annual Report for year ending January 30, 2010, http://issuu.com/actionfund/docs/ppfa_financials_2010_ 122711_web_vf?mode=window&viewMode=doublePage.

4. David Crary, "After Scandal, Foes Target Planned Parent-hood," Associated Press, February 14, 2011, http://www.msnbc .msn.com/id/41572487/ns/health-sexual_health/t/wake-scandal -foes-target-planned-parenthood.

5. Shaker Jane, "Chipping Away at Breast Healthcare," Shakesville .com, January 30, 2012, http://www.shakesville.com/2012/01/ chipping-away-at-breast-healthcare.html.

6. David Crary, "Planned Parenthood loses Komen funds," Associated Press, February 1, 2012, http://www.usatoday.com/USCP/PNI/ Nation/World/2012-02-01-APUSPlannedParenthoodKomen_ ST_U.htm.

7. Laura Bassett, "Komen Cuts Planned Parenthood Grants Months After Arrival Of New VP, Who Is Abortion Foe," HuffingtonPost .com, January 31, 2012, http://www.huffingtonpost.com/2012/ 01/31/komen-planned-parenthood-cuts-karen-handel_n_ 1245568.html.

8. Erin Gloria Ryan, "Disgrace For The Cure," Jezebel.com, January 31, 2012, http://jezebel.com/disgrace-for-the-cure/.

9. Glenn Gaudet, "Lessons from the Komen Controversy," Social MediaToday.com, February 7, 2012, http://socialmediatoday.com/ glenn-gaudet/441446/lessons-komen-controversy.

Chapter 8: Implosion

1. http://articles.businessinsider.com/2011–05–16/strategy/29979962_1_hazing-instructor-oral-exams; http://www.trainingmag.com/article/seven-steps-successful-murder-board.

2. *Morning Joe* (MSNBC), April 6, 2012.

3. "Head Of LA County's Susan G. Komen Chapter Tells CBS2 She's Resigning," CBS Los Angeles, February 2, 2012, http://losangeles.cbslocal.com/2012/02/02/head-of-la-countys-susan-g-komen-chapter-tells-cbs2-shes-resigning/.

4. http://www.propublica.org/special/komens-contortions-a-timeline-of-the-charitys-shifting-story-on-planned-par.

5. Laura Bassett, "Karen Handel, Susan G. Komen's Anti-Abortion VP, Drove Decision to Defund Planned Parenthood," Huffington Post.com, February 5, 2012, http://www.huffingtonpost.com/2012/02/05/karen-handel-susan-g-komen-decision-defund-planned-parenthood_n_1255948.html.

Chapter 9: Leaving Komen

1. Hilary Rosen, Twitter post, February 3, 2012, http://twitter.com/hilaryr.

2. Ibid.

3. http://www.lifenews.com/2012/02/17/komen-survey-still-considering-de-funding-planned-parenthood/.

Conclusion

1. Kirsten Powers, "Democratic Fears Fade as War on Women Wounds GOP," TheDailyBeast.com, April 18, 2012, http://www.thedailybeast.com/articles/2012/04/18/democratic-fears-fade-as-war-on-women-wounds-gop.html.

2. http://www.politico.com/blogs/burns-haberman/2012/07/polling
-memo-planned-parenthoods-antiromney-ads-leave-128311.html.

3. http://www.youtube.com/watch?v=60ziBFRKTnk.

4. Caroline May, "Pro-life group's hidden camera footage shows
complicity in 'sex-selective' abortions," DailyCaller.com, May 29,
2012, http://dailycaller.com/2012/05/29/pro-life-groups-hidden
-camera-footage-shows-complicity-in-sex-selective-abortions/.

5. Ibid.

6. Ben Shapiro, "The War on Unborn Women," Townhall.com, May
30, 2012, http://townhall.com/columnists/benshapiro/2012/05/30/
the_war_on_unborn_women.

7. Steven Ertelt, "Planned Parenthood Opposes Ban on Sex-Selection
Abortions," LifeNews.com, May 31, 2012, http://www.lifenews
.com/2012/05/31/planned-parenthood-opposes-ban-on-sex
-selection-abortions/.

8. Caroline May, "Obama opposes ban on sex-selective abortions,"
DailyCaller.com, May 31, 2012, http://dailycaller.com/2012/05/31/
obama-opposes-ban-on-sex-selective-abortions/.

9. "Susan G Komen NC Affiliate Names New Executive Director,"
WRAL-TV, http://www.wral.com/news/local/noteworthy/story/
11258224/.

10. Lynn Bonner, "North Carolina House passes budget after heated
debate," NewsObserver.com, May 30, 2012, http://www.news
observer.com/2012/05/30/2100767/north-carolina-lawmakers
-squabble.html; and "In New Abortion Battle, Planned Parenthood
Sues Arizona," Reuters, July 17, 2012; http://in.reuters.com/article/
2012/07/17/abortion-plannedparenthood-arizona-idINL2E8IH01
E20120717.

11. http://online.wsj.com/article/SB1000142405270230355210457743
8421678904222.html?mod=WSJ_Opinion_LEADTop.

12. http://www.lifenews.com/2012/06/05/networks-still-silent-on
-planned-parenthood-sex-selection-expose/.